HELP! MY BOOB IS SICK!

My Beautiful Mess With Cancer

Amanda Feliz
Lynn, Massachusetts

Copyright © 2025 by Amanda Feliz

All rights reserved.

No portion of this book may be reproduced in any form without written permission from the publisher or author, except as permitted by U.S. copyright law.

ISBN: 979-8-9995427-1-7 (Ebook)
ISBN: 979-8-9995427-0-0 (Paperback)
ISBN: 979-8-9995427-2-4 (Hardcover)

Library of Congress Control Number: 2025917492

Amanda Feliz
PO BOX 2623
Lynn, MA 01903

To contact the author, email her at Feliz_auth@proton.me.

I dedicate my story to my mom, Deborah, who passed away from pancreatic cancer, and to my stepdad, who passed away a year later from heartache. I know you are smiling down on me from the other side and are proud of me! I wish we had more time together on earth so I could share my desire to write a book about my journey and so much more. You were my biggest fan in life!

I also dedicate this book to anyone who is currently undergoing treatment. May you find hope, positivity, and peace for the days ahead!

Lastly, I dedicate this story to anyone who is dealing with a family member, friend, coworker, or other who has been diagnosed with the big C. May you find comfort and light in these pages!

Table of Contents

Welcome to My Beautiful Mess!	1
1. Life's Unexpected Paths	5
2. Cascading Mountains of Stress	31
3. The Worst Possible News	57
4. Facing a Harsh Reality	87
5. My Treatment Journey	119
6. To Hair or Not to Hair?	165
7. Ringing the Bell	185
Epilogue	207
Follow the Author	217
Practical Tips from an Overcomer	219

Acknowledgments	225
Resources	229
About the Author	235

Welcome to My Beautiful Mess!

♥

The day I got the diagnosis of breast cancer, everything shifted. The life I had worked so hard to create and the dreams I had set aside for some future time felt like they were fading away in that moment. Time froze, and I found myself in a long silence. The uncertainty and the fear of the unknown weighed on me heavily. I wondered, "Will I make it through? What physical and emotional changes am I about to face?"

As time went by, I gradually gained strength within me to go on. Cancer did not just test my body; it reached my very soul, forcing me to find courage I did not even know I had. In the midst of the pain, tears, sleepless nights, and never-ending treatments, there were always small moments of gratitude that helped me journey on.

My memoir is more than just a story of surviving breast cancer. It's about rediscovering how to truly live afterward, and it's also about moments of love and kindness that brought me joy on my saddest days. The acts of kindness and care gave me strength and courage while facing something so scary.

I share my story to let you and anyone else who might be going through a similar journey know that you are not alone. While this book is specifically about my breast cancer journey, unfortunately, we all deal with stress and struggle at some point in our lives. As I start out by explaining the very real struggles and stresses I was dealing with at the time, I hope it explains how I believe these things contributed to my diagnosis.

Most importantly, I hope you find your own healing for your own life, no matter the journey you are facing. There is always hope, even in the toughest times, and the possibility of new beginnings is always attainable!

Chapter 1
Life's Unexpected Paths

♥

"We must accept finite disappointment, but we must never lose infinite hope."
~ Martin Luther King, Jr.

My Winding Career Path

The year was 2010, and I was making a major career decision: it was time to quit working for Verizon. What a big deal for me! This job had been my financial stability for more than ten years, making it possible for me to provide for my two children like any good mom would do.

Thinking back to when I first began to consider working for Verizon, my long-term dreams were hanging in the balance. I was successfully employed at a local law firm at the time, and I didn't want to leave my current job. Yet, in looking over the Verizon contract, I knew that my children and I would be a lot better off financially by my switching paths. The promised salary increases every three months at Verizon would actually double my current salary from the law firm within a year's time!

Another incentive that prompted me to work at Verizon was their offer to pay for additional educational opportunities. I developed the perfect plan: give up my current employment in my desired industry and switch to Verizon so that I could enjoy financial stability while furthering my long-term career plans to immerse myself in the legal field. When I looked into all of the details, money was what drew me to Verizon, but I knew that it wasn't enough to keep me there forever. I had a dream to pursue.

All during the period I was employed at Verizon, I harbored thoughts about when I would start going to law school. The nagging urge to become a lawyeress had been incessant since childhood. Call it an infatuation if you will, but everything about the field of legalese and lawyering had always inspired me.

Part of this stemmed from the poverty I faced while growing up and getting the clear impression that lawyers make a lot of money, which I first remember realizing in 6th grade. I envisioned creating a better life for myself by working hard to become a lawyeress. Then, when I was 13, I had the opportunity to do a little under-the-table work for a local attorney, *wepa wepa*. She happened to deal with care and protection cases, so I was fascinated when reading the files and learning that she helped kids who were my age. By understanding legal cases from this close-up perspective, it was no longer just about making money. It finalized everything for me. *¡Qué bien!*

With such legal pursuits always having occupied my mind, I had a clear career path. Telecommunications was definitely not part of my *joie de vivre* but more of a means to an end. I already had my associate's degree in Legal Administrative Assistance. So, I took steps to earn my bachelor's degree and later enrolled in an educational program to get my paralegal certificate. These were easy decisions to make because Verizon was covering my educational expenses, and I was taking concrete steps to fulfill my dreams in the legal field. Unknown to me, that mystery thingy called fate or our true calling would have my plans turn out otherwise.

Then there was something Verizon offered from the beginning of my career with them that caught my eye: a severance package! The first time I heard corporate present the different options, I was like "What?? *¡Loco!* I need *mucho dinero*! Why would I leave?" BUT, I knew these packages were there for a reason, so I always kept that offering in the back of my mind.

I also noticed that corporate frequently offered severance packages while still regularly hiring more people every year, which gave me many opportunities to wonder about the direction of my career path. In looking around at my coworkers, I often thought that if I did not accept the package and leave sooner rather than later, then I would be stuck there forever.

"Get out while you're young," I told myself, and I know now that if I didn't leave when I did, then I would still be there today.

One time, I recall coming across the severance package and saying to myself, "Give me at least double that, and I will leave Verizon in a heartbeat and without a second thought!"

Little did I know, since I put that out into the universe, this exact opportunity would soon come my way. According to the law of attraction, when you put something out there, it will happen.

In this case, the significance for me was that when the package I had spoken into existence did come out, it was actually more than double! Just like I told myself, I didn't think about it twice. Here was my chance to make a decision and shift my course! I signed that severance package and walked!

So many people thought I was *loca* because I had children to support, but I had a bigger plan to pursue: obtain my paralegal certificate. The severance package would keep me financially secure while working toward my next career goal. For the people who first thought I was *loca en la cabeza* for leaving a good-paying job, the *mucho dinero* was all there. If they knew the details of that hefty severance package, I'm sure they would have thought that I was *loca* for NOT taking it!

I accepted Verizon's severance package in June, and I soon found out that I was in a whole line-up of people who were staggered to leave the company according to seniority. My exit date was now scheduled for September, so in the meantime, I had a lot of plans to make in regards to employment, education, and life in general.

I found out that if I was enrolled in school *before* I officially left, then Verizon would continue to cover those expenses! This was even better than I expected! I began taking a paralegal program on Saturdays shortly before my exit date in September, and I knew that Verizon would continue paying for my education so I could get my Paralegal Certificate. I felt that the future was set up in my favor.

With my goal of becoming an attorney newly sparked into action, I prepared further and took the LSATs. Then I sent applications to two reputable universities in MA, making sure to postmark both applications by the March 1st deadline. Not realizing how much work went into the applications, I was up all night before the deadline to complete the paperwork!

Looking back, I am certain that everything happens for a reason. While I thought that I had always wanted to be a lawyer, I realize now that if I truly wanted that career, I would have finished those applications weeks in advance. Plus, I didn't try my best on the LSAT because of everything in my personal life, including a messy divorce, but I still managed to get accepted to a waiting list. At the time, however, with my Verizon resignation in hand and my paralegal studies being paid for, I was content for the severance package to carry me forward until the next opportunity opened up.

Volunteering at the Library

On a sunny morning in September 2010, the aura of a quickly departing summer was still lingering in the air. I was dropping off my son Wesley for his first day of school when the school's librarian came up to me and told me that she was looking for parent volunteers.

"Okay, I'll do it!" I enthusiastically agreed. I was always looking for ways to be more involved in my kids' education, whether that meant joining the PTO or helping with other activities at their school. Here was just the kind of opportunity I was looking for! As I affirmatively told the librarian that I was absolutely interested in volunteering, I gave her the grin of a child who had just received the best Christmas present. *¡Qué emotion!*

I offered to go in every Monday morning, thinking to myself that I would treat volunteering like my real job by getting up early and having something to do. So, instead of going to work at Verizon, I began volunteering at the library where my son attended elementary school. My work consisted of helping the librarian with whatever she needed assistance with, which mostly meant putting away and organizing the books. Meanwhile, I continued my paralegal program on Saturdays through the end of the year.

While volunteering from September 2010 to February 2011, I developed a great network and made many friendships with different colleagues. Occasionally, they would jokingly nudge me to become a substitute teacher. I kept refusing, citing the fact that I was going to be attending law school soon and that my volunteer work was only temporary. I even told the principal about my intentions so that all of us were on the same page.

At the same time, I secretly enjoyed looking at the students' work on the bulletin boards as I walked through the hallways in my travels to and from the library. Even though my goals were still focused elsewhere, I was still curious about the teacher world. Every time I saw the littles walk the hallways, it brought me back to my days when I was a kid in school.

Meanwhile, I had already taken steps to immerse myself in the legal field by pursuing my paralegal certification studies. My unwavering intent to go to law school dictated that I *not* become a teacher, so I continued to resolutely remind others that I was content with simply being a volunteer.

Financial Woes

As the world turned, my personal life was in crisis. It had been two years since I had separated from my then-husband. I had gone through a devastating and draining divorce process, leaving me with a heavy burden of financial debt. I had been determined to end the marriage, and the financial burden was a price I was willing to pay, even if it meant working my ass off to pay off that accumulated debt.

My previous cry into the universe had been met and manifested itself when I received a hefty severance package from Verizon. Part of it came in a lump sum, and the remainder was spread out in monthly payments over the course of the next few years. This severance package guaranteed me financial peace for a while, and was especially handy for paying bills, marital debt, and tax arrears. I successfully continued to work hard to pay all my bills off and keep all the vexatious bill collectors at bay.

Six months later, however, I no longer had a steady source of income. It was inevitable that the reliable money from the severance package would begin to run low. You see, I owed a LARGE tax debt to the IRS and the Massachusetts Department of Revenue, which was foolishly incurred while I was still married due to a change in taxation withholding status. We had agreed that the cost would be split by both of us, but when the time came around to pay the taxes, he was gone. I was left high and dry, proving in retrospect that the earlier decision we had agreed upon was detrimental. *¡Lo peor que yo es hecho!*

A New Journey in Substitute Teaching

As a result of my financial situation becoming dire, the offer I received from my son's elementary school to become a substitute teacher suddenly became appealing. The staff continued to encourage me to give it a try, so I began the application process and contacted the school administration to inform them about my change of status. In response, they booked me as a substitute teacher for several days, even though the process was still ongoing and I had not yet been actually approved. Once I was officially hired, those tentative dates became a reality. *¡Qué alegria!* What happiness!

As word went around the district that taking a chance on me would be an excellent decision, two more schools besides my son's school began to regularly schedule me into their calendar. With substitute work being on an as-needed basis, I soon began juggling between the three schools. I was even scheduled at additional schools since there were a total of 18 different elementary schools in the district, all within a 20-minute commute.

Early in the morning, my phone would ring to inform me which school needed me that day, and off I would go on my new career adventure. I especially enjoyed working at my son's school since it was a convenient walk. Another nearby school was also particularly impressed with my abilities, not only with my work with the kids but also as a translator. At one point, they told me, "We don't know where you are working the rest of the year, but we are booking you for the rest of the year!" *¡Estaba tan agradecida!* Like, WOW!

Although the experience of working as a substitute teacher was great, I was being paid a measly $75 per day. This was far from enough to meet the cost of living for *me y mi familia*, my son Wesley and my daughter Angela. I was a single mother with no expectation of support from either father, so I had a lot to maintain for the three of us. After all, it is a well-known fact that it takes two incomes to maintain a household in America, with the primary reason being that the cost of living has not kept pace with the average salary.

Knowing that I needed to supplement my current income, I embarked on a job-searching mission. As fate would have it, I found an opportunity that looked perfect: an after-school job at the local YMCA. Since I was already working with kids at the elementary schools, it was even more advantageous to continue working with kids for the rest of each day! Best of all, my son was already attending a program at the Y, so once I was approved for the job, it was a bonus to see him throughout the afternoon and go home together when my work was done for the day.

Building Sub on the Horizon

As the months went by, I continued to maintain my busy substitute teacher's schedule. It was toward the end of the 2011 school year when the current principal at the elementary school approached me in the hallway one day. She expressed that the school was in a tight spot, particularly because they needed a building substitute. While she had already asked someone else, she wanted to see if I was on board as a possible back-up.

I had already learned the difference: a regular sub can get called into any school within the district every day, and a building sub is assigned to one particular school for the entire school year. While the building substitute position came with the additional requirements to show up for all 180 days of the school year and to help with miscellaneous tasks when not needed to replace a teacher, it also provided more permanence and a little bit more compensation as well. Instead of a measly $75 per day with the hopes of a phone call each morning, this was $100 a day with guaranteed work!

I replied in the affirmative, saying, "Absolutely!" I'm sure *mi contentemento y allegria* showed through.

After that conversation, and also in the days to follow, I began considering the two career paths before me. I had successfully received my paralegal certificate the prior December, but had not actively pursued working in a law firm. On the other hand, after making such a good first impression in the school district, I continued subbing into the New Year instead of seeking other employment. I realized that it was possible for me to become a teacher in this supposedly short period of life, so I decided to put aside my law school ambitions for the time being and focus on the best ways to support my family.

Soon, I found out that the other person whom the principal asked to be the building sub accepted the position, so I knew that it meant

I would not have that opportunity any longer. Fully content with that decision, I spent the summer feeling relaxed and contemplating my next moves. What would I do for the future? Continue substitute teaching for the local schools? Seek a position as a full-time paralegal or legal secretary?

While in this indecisive maze, I received a phone call from the elementary school principal out of the blue. She informed me that while the other candidate had taken the job, there was one important detail they had initially missed that made her no longer qualified for the position. The job was once again offered to me!

I was elated by the prospect of being the building sub! I already enjoyed the job of a substitute teacher, and I would be working every day in the same location. I also knew that this would make a little more money, a guaranteed

$100 per day. Plus, it was so convenient and just a three-minute walk from my house!

While excited about my increased salary, practically speaking, I knew that the building sub money was still not enough for our family of three. So, as the new school year began, I continued to supplement my income with my secondary job as an after-school counselor at the YMCA. How convenient it was to be in the same building as my son, both at school every day and at the Y afterward as well!

Looking back, I often wonder how I felt a sense of relief at my new building sub salary being a mere $500 per week. How did we survive?? I remember one thing for certain: my stress levels were very high during this time of life as I balanced two jobs and took care of my two children. Around the same time, I also made the decision to stop smoking pot after using that habit occasionally over the years to maintain a sense of calm and comfort in my life. Little did I know at the time, the stress surrounding these coinciding events would soon lead to the greatest challenge of my life.

Conflict at the YMCA

At some point during the school year, I was involved in a minor accident when someone bumped into my car. I was perfectly okay, but I desperately needed my vehicle to be repaired since it was my only means of transportation.

On a typical day, I worked from 7:45 AM to 2:00 PM as a building sub. Immediately after, I would proceed to the YMCA to get ready for the kids to show up at 2:30 PM, where we all would stay until 6:00 PM. Consequently, I had no time for appointments. I knew that the brief half-hour between the end of the school day and the beginning of the after-school program afforded me no time to go get car repairs done or to acquire a rental car as a temporary vehicle while leaving my car at the shop.

I proceeded to talk to the YMCA management about my situation. I let them know that I needed to come in late for my next shift on one particular day to deal with the urgent car repair. Unfortunately, the managerial staff were not as empathetic as I had hoped they would be, and they declined to accommodate my unforeseen circumstance. *Okay, ¡esta bien!*

Worst of all, their attitude really pissed me off. "*¡Qué mierda!*" I thought. "Here I am, a grown-ass woman with two children and two jobs, and they don't give me any slack! It's time to reevaluate my life. Anyway, they are my side gig, not my main gig!"

At that point, I asked the YMCA to cut back my hours to three days a week so I could handle various matters for my family during my free afternoons. Unsurprisingly, they were uncooperative, even after adamantly denying me my time-off request the first time. So, I handled my car situation by telling them that I would be in a bit later than usual on a particular day to handle my grown folk business at the car rental place. I didn't even ASK for the whole day off. Instead, I TOLD them what I would be doing.

Next, I began looking for a different part-time job that would better accommodate my busy life. Since I was familiar with another program that Angela attended called Girls Inc., I applied for a job there. I told them that my availability was three afternoons a week, and I was soon accepted. Success! ¡Qué alegría!

Consequently, I explained to Wes that I wasn't going to be working at the after-school program with him anymore. While disappointed, he understood. As soon as I was accepted at Girls Inc., I gave the YMCA my two-week notice and prepared for the transition between jobs. As I looked forward to the future, my biggest hope was that my life and its many responsibilities would become much more manageable. *Que Dios me acompañe en mi decisión.*

"Hope is necessary in every condition. The miseries of poverty, of sickness, or captivity would, without this comfort, be insupportable."
~ Samuel Johnson

Chapter 2

Cascading Mountains of Stress

♥

"It is a mistake to look too far ahead. Only one link of the chain of destiny can be handled at a time."
~ Winston Churchill

My History with Stress

All my life, I have dealt with an inordinate amount of stress. My years of experience as a teacher and my daily opportunities to observe the lives of kids under my care have only served to open my eyes further to this fact. Yet, my newfound awareness is no longer just about facing my own stress. Instead, I use it to stay extremely aware of what my students are dealing with in their own lives.

For instance, if we gain a new student and I find out that they're in their third school or going to therapy, I am extraordinarily empathetic toward them. Also, if any of my students leave without saying goodbye, I remember how I went through that very same kind of circumstance in my childhood. Even though I don't know their exact situation, if one of my students leaves abruptly, I try to find out where they went and give them their papers to help them on their new journey and provide them with some closure.

Thinking back to the hardships of my own childhood, I have a lot of new insight when remembering those days through my adult eyes. Ever since I was little, I would face stressors that caused me to feel disappointed and sad. For example, my mom was a single mom and had to work a lot, so when I was little and living with my mom, I often had to stay with different babysitters. I also grew up feeling that I was always activated, either in fight or in flight mode. I learned to smile regardless of my struggles, but it was very difficult and not something that anyone should have to deal with their whole life.

I would occasionally visit my dad and enjoyed visiting him, but those times were stressful as well. Each time I would go back home to my mom, I was forced to ask the question, "When will I see Dad again?"

Additionally, at the end of every visit, I was told to go into my house to change. I was always expected to take off whatever clothes I had been wearing while at my dad's and give them back to whoever dropped me off. I hated doing this! *¡Qué vergüenza!*

The story I was always given was that I had to change clothes because my mom didn't take care of me or my stuff, but that didn't make sense. To me as a kid, all I understood was that I had play clothes and school clothes, and I knew that I would get in trouble if I was caught playing while wearing school clothes.

As I grew older, I spent a lot of time moving around, being shuffled between family members, and navigating new schools with every move. I couldn't wait to grow up and be old enough to move out!

When I was 17, I graduated from high school in early June and moved out of my aunt's house within a week. My family said that I ran away, but I intentionally left, *Jesus santisimo*. I guess it sounds like the same thing, but it really depends on who you talk to. The truth of the story, if you want to get down to it, is that my family basically kicked me out.

I was finally free! My family wanted me to move out and go live with my mom in another town, but I had a job and a boyfriend in Lynn, so that's where I wanted to stay. Since I was over 17, I figured out my next move on my own and made it. It didn't help that I was hard-headed! Immediately upon moving out, and for several months after, I decided not to talk to my family but deal with life on my own. I always managed to figure it out!

Being in another environment was a whole NEW kind of stress and its own hot mess. I had no idea what I was about to find out, but I soon learned all about dealing with the DCF and foster homes and the entire lifestyle that went with it. These were things that I had only heard about since my family was very church-oriented, and we always tried to be very respectful of each other by keeping everything within our own family. Suffice it to say that this is a different long story for another day!

I had my daughter Angela when I was young, and we were supported by welfare at first, which helped me get an apartment and a job at a law firm. *¡Gracias a Dios!* I eventually got my associate's degree in Legal Administrative Assistance as well, and then I was able to be more independent with a new job as a legal secretary for a law firm. Rent was also a lot cheaper in those days, so I was able to keep my own place.

Overall, I faced a lot of stress on my own, but I soon learned that you just have to keep smiling even though you're stressed. I had to find happiness in my challenging life. Otherwise, I would always be miserable. That's just part of life, and I had to do the best that I could do. As I like to say, grin, bear it, and find your joy!

As I dealt with every situation back-to-back, the stress became intertwined so strongly with my life to the point where I finally realized that I didn't know what a stress-free life was. I only knew chaos! Even now, as weird as it may be, I recognize that if I don't have any stress or chaos in my life, then I'm creating some! I do try to clear it, but sometimes it seems like I can't get out of my own way.

Another thing I've learned is that as stressful things in my life build up, it's the growth past such challenges that makes it worth it. No matter how extremely hard the chaos may feel at times, I look at each day as it comes. *¡Eso es la vida!*

Often, stress and chaos are like an invisible wall. Even though you can't see it, it's still there, building up pressure like a volcano and constantly knocking at your door. That's why it's so important to deal with all of the little yucky stuff so it doesn't blow up and create a worse problem! I can often tell that I'm having a hard time when the little stress button in the back of my mind starts to grow bigger, triggered by basic things like looking for something I need. I try to handle it the best I can by living each day with minimal stress and then taking little steps to find healing from my own trauma.

Since living with stress or chaos is just the way my life has been dealt to me, I can't mope and cry about it. I have embraced it as being part of who I am and looked to keep a positive attitude no matter what. All I can do is just take life as it comes, hope that it gets better, and try to be a better person every day. Keep it movin'!

My Teaching Schedule

With that backdrop in mind, life was no different when I started my new job as a building sub. Daily stress was just part of the package! Every morning, I would wake up early to get my kids ready for school and prepare myself for work. Wes was nine years old and in elementary school, while Angela was seventeen years old and in high school. Every morning was rushed, every day was full for each of us, and every evening we would come back together as a family and try to connect before going to sleep and waking up to do it all over again.

In my role as a parent, I had to make sure that Wes was doing his homework and Angela was doing well in school and not failing. As a good mom, I was always paying attention to each one of their needs, from their clothes to their moods.

Since I was working two jobs, I had very little time for necessary tasks like setting up dentist and doctor appointments and taking care of bills, grocery shopping, cooking, cleaning, and other adult responsibilities. As a result, these tasks would build up. Yet, if I missed one job so I could prioritize home life over work and attend to any one of my obligations, then money would be adjusted, which only served to stress me out even more. I was already struggling to make ends meet!

In the school environment, which was my main job, I was very heavily focused on the school day. I took notes while making observations of other staff in different classes, recognizing the things that I liked so I could eventually implement them in my own classroom. Working as a sub was really like "playing teacher," since I had no lesson plans and did my best to figure out how to develop my skills as an instructor.

With no formal education in the field that I had recently jumped into, I was also required to take my MTELs (Massachusetts Teacher Equivalency Lesson Tests) to receive the necessary teacher license and then qualify for better teaching positions. I was doing my best to study for and schedule tests so I could advance my education and my job status.

Since I already had my bachelor's, all I needed to do was pass each required test. From there,

I would get my preliminary five-year license, and then I could advance the license to initial by getting my master's in education. I was also exploring other alternatives that would fit into my lifestyle.

Meanwhile, due to my work schedule, both of my children attended after-school programs. Wes, in particular, had attended after-school daycare since preschool so I could work full-time. Once I transitioned from two jobs down to just one teaching job, Wes started hanging out with me after school and no longer required after-school care.

In addition to all of our daily home, school, and work responsibilities, both of my kids had several extracurricular activities. Angela focused on dance, gymnastics, swimming, track, and basketball. Wesley played baseball and basketball. When she was younger, Angela was also involved in weekly activities at the Catholic Church and went through classes to take her first communion. Both Angela and I went to therapy at the time, so that was an added obligation on top of our already full schedules.

Throughout our stressful days, weeks, months, and years, one assuaging factor was that I kept in touch with both of my children throughout each day. This helped me avoid feeling like I was being an absentee parent and really helped soften the blow. Since the time Angela was in middle school, for instance, I would take the time every day to get in touch with her by cell phone to learn her whereabouts and see how she was doing.

Getting home between 6:30 PM and 7:00 PM on school days brought other challenges. As can be imagined, I was already worn out from a long day's work, but I had my unpaid and critically essential jobs at home waiting for me every day.

First, I would have to figure out an answer to the question that I never quite could nail down: "What's for dinner?" Dinner options were not an easy choice, so on most occasions, I would forgo cooking because it was time-consuming and getting late, often resorting to quick fixes that would allow me to pop something into the microwave or oven while sitting down to check if my son was doing his homework. We often settled for leftovers, pizza, cheap and processed frozen dinners, or greasy and fatty takeout. My goal was to make sure my kids were eating as many healthy, well-rounded meals as possible, but since they both loved whatever crap we ended up eating, I didn't feel too guilty as a busy mom for not having better options.

In the next lineup of mommy duties, I had to make sure both of my kids finished their homework, showered, and got ready for bed. As they grew older and took more responsibility for themselves, I still had to make sure they were both in bed on time and not having too much screen-time. Of course, if either of them stepped out of line, I needed to discipline them as well.

Most of all, I did my best to protect both of my kids from stress, putting all of it on my own shoulders as any good mother would do. As a result, I continued to gain weight, often fluctuating between eating nothing and eating everything in sight. I kept thinking that what I was eating was not good for my health. Nevertheless, while dealing with daily stressors, I continued to gain more and more weight, telling myself that I must stop this pattern before I ended up on the extreme end of the sick spectrum. Unfortunately, since I often told myself that my habits were going to get me very sick, all I was doing was practicing the law of attraction by putting that thought out there.

My work schedule being what it was, it literally felt like I was stuck in a bad trap. I got up early, went to job one, then went to job two, came home late, was too tired to eat well, and the cycle went on and on. I became increasingly taxed both mentally and physically. I needed the two jobs financially but was quickly wearing myself down. *Señor, ten piedad.*

Effectively, I was in a quandary. I was extremely stressed with my life circumstances. I was tired all the time, I had no time to cook, I was financially strapped, and I was trying to take care of my kids and household chores. Given my propensity to gain weight, I gained so much weight during that time that it was depressing. To rub salt on my injuries, my financial situation was as tumultuous and distressful as could be, to say the least, despite working two jobs. It was a constant and unrelenting struggle as I tried to keep up with all my financial obligations. *Ave Maria, purísima que voy hacer.*

Psychosomatic Expression

Since the mind and body are deeply connected, real physical symptoms arise from and are influenced by mental patterns. I really believe there is a powerful mind-body connection because of how I inwardly knew and could foresee that I was going to face extreme ill health if I stayed on my current trajectory. Yet, it was extremely difficult to exercise any kind of self-discipline in the area of eating. Food made me feel so much better because it was so yummy and comforting! I knew that if I didn't stop, I would get very sick—not a regular kind of sick but a very serious kind of sick!

In fact, weight had always been an issue for me because of my tendency to comfort myself through food, though it was easier to lose weight when I was younger. This pattern started out in my childhood since I did not have a strict diet when I was with my mom. At Mom's, I often ate hot dogs, bologna, ramen, and similar unhealthy foods. After the age of seven, I moved to Dad's, where we constantly ate rice and beans, which really helped pack on the pounds!

As I grew older, it became normal to gain and lose weight. I would recognize my weight issue, focus on losing, and shed 80 pounds. Then I would turn around and gain some more before focusing on losing again and shedding, say, 60 pounds. Food was always so comforting and yummy!

The pattern of gaining and losing finally reached a breaking point when I was getting my master's in education. I realized that I had more control over my relationship with food. I told myself that I *could* eat a whole plate of food, but that would only result in me going comatose. So, I would literally cut my meal in half, eat one portion to satisfy my hunger, and then save the rest for another yummy meal! I could not afford to eat the whole meal because there was a lot of pressure to get work done instead of spending a lot of time eating large meals and sleeping. This time around, it worked more naturally, except when it came to McDonald's French fries!

The Discovery

Somewhere deep inside of me, I knew that I needed to permanently control my weight to remain healthy. Still, I was in denial and progressively became obese. I discovered that when you are obese, you especially avoid looking at your naked self, so I took the extra effort to avoid seeing the woman in the mirror I had become.

I was ashamed of that woman! I was only able to muster enough courage to look at myself in the mirror while accoutered in some of my best garbs. My clothes masked the reality of my obesity to my visual senses a little bit, but I was unable to mask the reality in my mind. Yet, as much as I avoided looking at my naked self in the mirror, it's a fact of life that it must happen, and it happens often.

So, in one of those moments of undress, I took a closer look at the sight in the mirror. *Pero, pero y eso.*

"What in God's green earth is that? *¡Ay Dios mío!*" I took a step toward the mirror and then moved a step back. Then I took a step even closer and made a more careful observation of my left breast.

"WTF!" I exclaimed. "What's wrong with my boob? WTF!"

My nipple was pulled in, and there was a little line where my nipple normally popped out. I had never seen my nipple like that. For just a second, it brought me back to that prepubescent period when waiting for the nipple to develop.

"Did I put on so much weight that my boobs are weird and funny now?" was one of the many questions that conjured in my mind. I knew that gaining an inordinate amount of weight concurrently alters your physical appearance, so maybe that was it.

To be honest, I was a little mean to myself, deciding to follow up the serious question with harsh criticism. "Look at what you did to yourself, you fat bitch!"

At the same time, I wondered if there was something else going on altogether. It was a secret and nagging thought that I did my best to deny while secretly being afraid that it was already true.

I immediately did a manual breast exam, and I found a lump. Was it only fatty tissue? Or was it much worse? My deep, deep thought was that I had found a shameful, sad reality for myself after already warning myself repeatedly that by overeating, I was going to make myself very sick. That bad, chemical-ridden food had got me!

I tried not to be hard on myself, but growing up with a taste for unhealthy foods to help deal with all that childhood stress had continued down a dangerous path to the place I was now. A fresh urgency struck me, and I decided to act upon my weight. If I could only get to the gym regularly, take more steps throughout the day, and stick to a healthy diet, I would see the pounds start to diminish. I had done this before!

However, my daily schedule was already too overwhelming: two children to parent, two full-time jobs, required classes and exams to obtain a Massachusetts Teacher's Education license, and now I had to fit in a workout schedule! I was just one week away from the beginning of the new school year, and my life already had too many moving components. How was I going to add anything else to it?

As I stepped away from the mirror, reality struck. My plan to lose weight never materialized. My breast was not looking right, and it scared me, but I didn't want to think the worst. The denial was real and it was heavy! I tried to calm my nervousness and anxiety by ignoring my reality and suppressing any thoughts that came up. I didn't even take the time to further explore the lump because a mix of realities was manifesting. I was a single mom and about to start a brand-new career as a first-year teacher. My kids needed me, and I needed to figure out teaching to make more money.

After all, I finally could see the end of the tunnel after leaving Verizon and being forced to work two jobs to make ends meet. If I could just survive this next phase of learning what it meant to be a teacher, then we would be more financially secure. Life would finally begin to settle down, and then I could focus on my weight, my health, and everything else I was currently ignoring.

Unfortunately, when you're finally forced to take note of the things that you have been ignoring for too long, you'll find them lurking out in the open, and it's never a good lurk.

"Hope is like the sun, which, as we journey toward it, casts the shadow of our burden behind us."
~ Samuel Smiles

Chapter 3

The Worst Possible News

♥

"Accept the things to which fate binds you, and love the people with whom fate brings you together, but do so with all your heart."
~ Marcus Aurelius, *Meditations*

New Career Paths

Despite all the pressure and stress I had been going through the whole year, I soldiered through and eventually obtained my preliminary teacher's license. This was a glimmer of sunshine on otherwise cloudy days! I had reason to be joyful and optimistic at the prospect of advancing from a building sub to a real classroom teacher. My two years of being a substitute teacher were finally coming to an end.

When I delivered the good news to the principal, she proceeded to offer me a chance to continue being a building sub for the upcoming school year. Accepting that offer would have defeated the purpose of obtaining my new teaching license, so I gently declined in anticipation of overseeing my own class. Of course, she knew that would be my response, so she told me about a teaching position that would be available in September.

Meanwhile, I was not only giving up but completely steering clear of my old lawyering dream. After having more recently dealt with various legal situations, including restraining orders, court cases, and more, I was left with a bad taste in my mouth. So, in comparison to the very sad and messed-up situations that took place in the courtroom, I found substituting and teaching very rewarding. I interacted with kids all day and found the classroom atmosphere to be lighthearted and fun. Now, with my official teacher's license in hand, I was happy to throw out the lawyering idea for good.

As I focused on being a teacher, some of my fondest memories from my earliest years came back to me. I remembered playing school with my stuffed animals! I would take all the extra or unused pages from my workbooks that were sent home with me, plus any other papers the teachers gave away. Then I would set them all up in front of my teddy bears and hold class. Some of my "students" gave me answers that had me using my red pen on the whole sheet—wrong!

wrong! wrong!—but some of them got it right. Now, I was thrilled to have a real job where I went off to play real school with real kids every day!

Lingering Illness

As we entered the fall season and the school year was in full swing, I caught a cold that seemed to linger for longer than usual. Even after I finally recovered, less than two weeks later, I fell ill from yet another persistent cold. This happened several times in a row, and I began to feel seriously perplexed about what exactly was going on with my health. I had always been a healthy person, so why could I not shake this cold?

In the middle of falling sick an awful number of times, the keen awareness of one of my colleagues was triggered. I remember her remarking, "Oh, you've been getting sick a lot this year. It's probably because of your new class and building up your immunity!"

I responded, "No, I should be over that by now." After all, I had been a building sub at the same school for two years, which meant that I had been constantly going in and out of classrooms every day and had already been exposed to many germs. My immune system should have been especially robust! If I had ever been a prime candidate for colds and flus, it was during my tenure as a building sub, not when I was stationed in a single classroom like I was now. So, it did not make sense to me that I was getting sicker now that I was only in one classroom. Even during past flu seasons, I had never gotten sick like I was currently suffering.

The only other clue that kept coming back to me was my level of stress. Everything had been slowly developing over the past couple of years when I was subbing and continued to grow over the summer. As I mentioned before, the increase in stress also coincided with my decision to stop smoking marijuana, which had served to be a major stress reliever for much of my adult life. Now, even though I was in just one classroom and beginning to see a light at the end of the stress tunnel, I was getting sick more often than when I had been exposed to hundreds of kids! Something strange was definitely going on.

That whole fall, I felt off. On Halloween, it was rainy and cold, and I was very tired. I felt my already limited energy going down and could tell that another cold was coming on, so I bribed Wes to stay home instead of taking him trick-or-treating. I offered to buy him a big bag of whatever candy he wanted along with a new video game from GameStop, and he very happily agreed. So, after hitting those two stores, we went home and curled up in bed for the rest of the night.

The following month during the Thanksgiving holiday, I worked around the clock to grade papers and create lesson plans. Even during the family meal, I had two tables set up near me and worked like a dog to get everything done over my break. My family couldn't believe it! As the first educator in my family, I often felt overwhelmed from working so hard to get through my first year of teaching. Plus, as an English language teacher, I was in my own little world.

Then, one December morning, I was unable to have a regular bowel movement. *¡Ay, ay, ay, que mierda!* Literally! This was highly unusual. Additionally, I was semi-constipated, and I rarely experienced constipation.

Consequently, alarm bells began clanging in my head. Something was terribly off, and I knew it.

In fact, I had already been realizing this about myself as the end of the year approached.

Soon, Christmas break was at hand. As all of us teachers left for recess, I was determined to use that whole break to rest. I needed my health to be restored! At the end of the holiday recess, however, I was only back at work for one day before calling out sick. Much to my dismay, my energy levels were on the low end of the spectrum and the bugging cold was back with me again, even after an extended break! It was the very first time since commencing my role as a new teacher that I contemplated calling out sick, and I finally did because I felt so poorly, but I was left feeling extremely guilt-ridden as a result.

My Daughter's Traumatic Experience

There was another part of my life that was also unraveling at the seams, creating another enormous day-to-day stressor. It's those background thoughts that stress you out, causing you to be genuinely concerned and haunting your every waking moment. More specifically, I had an ongoing legal issue pertaining to my daughter that was very traumatic and distressful, and it debilitated me with apprehension.

During the period following my departure from Verizon, I had much more free time that I mostly spent at home. During this period, my daughter Angela felt safe to confide in me many deeper things. Then, on one particular day, she delivered some devastating news while we were out driving. Her information shocked me to the bone, and I had to stop driving just to gather myself. After my heartbeat settled back down to near normal, I was able to compose myself, and we drove back home.

I was not prepared for the kind of news that my daughter had told me! Angela's revelation brought me unenviable exasperation mixed with trepidation. I cried my eyes out every night, I was constantly insomniac and could hardly sleep, and I had no energy to go to work so I could pay my bills. Yet, I tried my absolute best to conceal my visible despondency from my kids. As I dealt with my daughter's news, I was forced to try and face our day-to-day life the best I could and keep things running smoothly.

At the same time, my kids and I were close in our tiny apartment, so they noticed when I was in my room a lot and when I wasn't eating with them. They saw that it was hard for me to smile, have fun with them, and laugh the way we used to. I would make excuses when they wondered why I wasn't eating, so I would tell them that I had already eaten with friends. My kids would ask me if I was okay or if everything was all right, and as much as I tried to keep up a happy facade, they still knew deep down inside that something was going on.

Our routine did change ever so slightly, as I became a bit more relaxed about homework and occasionally became more tense about silly things like a mess in their bedroom. Everything felt like it began to be the opposite of what was normal, like maybe their room was tidy and there was a mess in the living room. Yet, I often had the attitude that I didn't care.

It was an uphill effort to mask my tribulations. I would go out, buy French fries, throw half of them out, and bring the rest back to my children. I would tell them that I had eaten enough and could not eat any more, when the reality was that I hadn't eaten at all. They did not see me eat for an extended period, but I did not want them to get concerned.

This went on for almost a month. I hardly ate a substantial meal or slept much at all, and all the while I was crying constantly. My stress levels were extremely high, and it was a miracle that I could even function!

At one point, I had a deeper conversation with Angela about the matter. As it turned out, the situation was reported, and the legal wheels took it from there. The District Attorney's office was regularly trying to contact me by phone to update me on the legal proceedings, arrange for a pre-trial, and schedule other miscellaneous meetings.

Visit to the General Practitioner

Meanwhile, I knew it was time to get some answers about my health, so I scheduled an appointment with my doctor. She was a general practitioner who encouraged me to remain optimistic about how I was doing overall, especially since she had been seeing me periodically over the past year for other issues and prescribing Lorazepam to help with my stress levels and sleep deprivation.

When I first mentioned my discovery of the lump, my doctor initially told me not to worry about it. In hindsight, she should have told me to worry so I would address my health and weight gain sooner! Yet, at the same time, she was focused on helping me face anxiety and depression due to all of the different situations in my life and did not want to cause me additional hardship.

On this visit, I expressed my worrisome discovery to my doctor in more detail—the retracted nipple and the lump in my breast. She examined my breast and was reassuring once again, hinting that it was probably nothing to worry about. At the same time, she recommended a further checkup and promptly proceeded to make an urgent diagnostic appointment for me at Salem Hospital.

The idea of a further checkup was unsettling! I set aside the specific day in February to address my health concerns and more recent scare. As it was the beginning of winter break, I was hopeful that I would have enough time to take care of all of my health issues at once and then be done with it by the time I finished the appointment and went back to work.

I left my doctor's office with an aura of nervousness and anxiety, the fear of the unknown lurking heavily on my mind. As the day of my appointment at Salem Hospital approached, I became increasingly nervous. I couldn't even sleep the night before in anticipation of what was to come. Many questions swirled through my mind. What if something was really wrong? What could I do then? God be with me! *Ay, que Dios me acompaña.*

Salem Hospital

It was February break in 2014, and the time for my appointment at Salem Hospital arrived. I had a particular dislike for this institution due to previous bad experiences while receiving services at their facilities that left a lingering bad taste in my mouth. Lo and behold, on this Tuesday morning, it was no different. Salem Hospital did not disappoint in disappointing me!

I arrived at the Breast Health Center at 8:15 AM, 15 minutes early for my appointment, only for the receptionist to adamantly inform me with an air of indifference, "You're late!"

"No, I am not late," I retorted with firm certitude. "My appointment is at 8:30 AM."

The receptionist apathetically and relentlessly continued to repeat that I was late, at which point I left the lobby, went back out to my car, and called my doctor's office.

As I sat in the parking lot waiting for the return phone call, I felt full of disbelief that I had been turned away from an appointment that I not only needed and anticipated but had even set the entire day aside for out of my excruciatingly busy schedule.

In the back of my mind, I had a worrisome inkling of a thought that I had been ignoring something serious about my health, so I was here to get it checked out. I planned to use part of my February vacation to address my health concerns, so I had the idea that this ordeal would only take a week. Thus, the reason for my great frustration.

My doctor called me right back, and I told her exactly what had just transpired while further explaining my resulting frustration at being turned away. Upon looking over the records, my doctor explained that, for some unknown reason, Salem Hospital set up two separate appointments for me—but that I was still on time for them. As a solution, she offered to send me to Massachusetts General Hospital (MGH) in Danvers instead. Luckily for me, they had an availability that morning.

I gladly left the inconsiderate Salem Hospital and drove straight to MGH. I was hopeful, thinking that I would still be able to focus on fixing my boob that day! As I found out later, Salem Hospital was reported for causing the unfortunate mix-up, so they sent me a letter some time afterward, apologizing for my inconvenience.

Massachusetts General Hospital

On the way to MGH, I called my mother to give her a heads-up about the change of plans. I shared my experience at Salem Hospital with her, since we often joked about how inept people at different businesses couldn't figure out how to simply do their own jobs. It was a nice moment between my mom and me to lighten the mood of the day ahead.

At the same time, I remembered the initial conversation that I had with my mother when I first discovered the lump. It was heart-wrenching to have to relay this sad news to my mother, and it was emotionally agonizing for both of us. I was distraught, and she was so sad that she cried for me. She had asked me at the time if she could accompany me to the appointment, but I had told her that I was just going to have a mammogram, which wouldn't take long. I believed that I would be fine, so I decided not to make a big deal out of it and left my friends and colleagues out of the developing circumstances until I had definitive test results.

I arrived at my appointment at MGH, and the receptionist was extremely nice—a welcome contrast from my treatment at Salem Hospital! She also told me I should not have been turned away from the original appointment, confirming my frustration with that other institution.

Then, a lovely nurse brought me into a private room and began asking me about my familial history of cancer. I was uncomfortably nervous answering these questions, knowing that there was indeed a record of cancer—both my father and grandfather had a past diagnosis of lymphoma. As I shared the history, I just held onto a hope deep down inside that these details were just a little blip in the family line and that everything was going to be fine.

After that, I had a mammogram done and entered the dreaded waiting period. The staff told me the doctor was in and would read the results right away, which was a surprise to me. I wasn't sure how normal it was at the time, so I thought to myself, "OMG! Why is the doctor reading it right away?"

Intuitively, I was aware that a positive cancer diagnosis was not far-fetched, but I chose to be in denial and avoided putting that vibe out there. It was extremely difficult to put that idea at bay, since the thought kept coming back like a flood of water that won't stop rushing. It was awful!

As I awaited the mammogram results, I was nervous, cold, and sweaty. Minutes felt like an eternity, and I felt like I had been there all day. I could feel myself slowly... slipping... into shock as I sat in the waiting room.

Finally, the medical staff came back! I felt like everything was in slow motion as a nurse told me that I would need a biopsy for further testing. Once again, they began asking me questions about my family history, and I struggled to answer as my mind raced.

"OMG! *¡Jesus santisimo!*" I thought. "I need my mother to know what is happening!" I was *en shock,* and that made reality hit a lot harder. The only other thing that came to mind was a prayer, "Give me strength in these moments! *¡Dame fuerza en estos momentos!*"

As the waves of cold continued to wash over me, the caring nurse told me that everything would be okay. Then the staff began bringing me warm blankets to combat the chills—the absolute best! They were the first of many warm blankets in the days to come. I had no idea that this was to be my new life, but I thank God for those warm blankets! *¡Gracias a Dios!* Those warm blankets carried me like nobody's business!!!

The Diagnosis

Two days after my mammogram, I had an appointment at the District Attorney's office. It was still February vacation from school, so my children went with me. After checking in at the office, I sat in the waiting room. I was making an effort to be happy and jolly with Angela and Wes as much as I could be, considering all of the circumstances for our being there in the first place and the other daunting thought about my health.

While waiting to be called into the office, I received a phone call from MGH in Danvers. "Here comes the mood killer!" I thought to myself. Naturally, I am dramatic, but I had good reason to be apprehensive, given the prospect of what the news was likely to be.

In fact, I was almost certain that it was not good news, and thus I could not help but start crying as I prepared to answer the phone. I took many deep breaths as I picked up the call, feeling my heart in my throat and a knot in my stomach as I continued to cry. Admittedly, I do make mountains out of mole hills, but this was certainly a mountain that I did not have to make bigger than what it really was!

On the other end of the line, it was the nice nurse who had met with me previously at the hospital. She did not hesitate to break the news to me but came straight out and told me the awful information.

"You have breast cancer."

I felt shocked by how abrupt it sounded, wondering if the nice part where a kind practitioner gently tells a patient about their cancer diagnosis only happens in the movies! I always had the attitude to brace myself for the worst and hope for the best. At that point, however, there was nothing else I could do except feel engulfed by sad emotions and immediately start bawling.

With my kids sitting right there beside me, I quickly became a crying mess. The whole DA's office was clouded in a quiet and awkward silence.

At the same time, in the middle of being very upset, I was not as shocked as I could have been. That deep, dark lurking sense that had been in my mind for some time, the one I kept fighting to push away and had ignored from the beginning, was finally being brought to light. I still had to try my best and be positive.

Like anything else that's inevitable, I had a choice: either go through the motions or make the best of it. For me, acknowledgement was the first step, even as I kept taking deep breaths to face the crushing anxiety. The more I accepted the unacceptable news, I knew it would be for the better. So, I chose to make the best of it, no matter what that looked like, because I knew there would be hard days ahead.

My major fear in these initial moments was realizing that I was going to deal with a lot of stuff that I probably would not want to. I knew the lump was big! I knew the journey ahead would be hard! Worst of all, I would have to tell my kids about my prognosis and try to hold it together for all three of us.

Before I had time to process further, the DA's office was calling me in. I remember walking down the hall, thinking to myself about how truly sad the situation was.

"Here I am at the DA's office, dealing with something huge that I am in the middle of!" I thought to myself. "As if that's not enough, now here comes another terrifying and life-altering issue!"

The reality was that I now had two battles to fight, and I had to win both of them. WTF!!! *Ruega por me, Santo Dio, cuidame.* Pray for me, God, and take care of me!

Honestly, I knew that all of the court shit was already big enough. Now, I was facing something truly major. I had my life to battle for!

All of these thoughts rushed through my mind as I walked down the hall. Just before I stepped into the office, I had one final question flash through my mind, "When do people break—and what is *my* breaking point?"

Once in the office, the staff could see the distress written all over my face. They asked me if everything was okay.

"No, it's not," I told them as I began to cry again. "I just got a phone call informing me that I have been diagnosed with breast cancer."

The staff immediately expressed their condolences, and we all remained silent for a moment out of respect for the somber and sad news. They then inquired if I was aware of how long treatments would likely take, and I told them that I didn't know. The only thing I could say for certain was that I had an appointment coming up, at which time I would find out more details.

The DA asked me to let them know as soon as possible so that they could try to postpone the legal proceedings until after the end of the treatments. I agreed to contact them once I had that information. I was there for a pre-trial meeting, but now all of this was to be postponed. Ouch!

As I left the DA's office, I was both happy and sad that they decided to postpone the proceedings and prioritize both me and my treatments. I was happy because I had a break in this area of life, but I was also sad because I like things to be resolved on the faster side. Now, this issue would be dragged out longer than it already had been!

Even with those dark thoughts, I was hopeful that something in my life could be fixed in just one day. Maybe those hopeful thoughts existed because I was still in denial, but I was simply relieved that I would be able to have the time to focus on whatever was coming my way next. More than that, I was happy that I found out what was wrong with me. Now the never-ending colds and constipation suddenly made sense!

> **"Life is a series of natural and spontaneous changes. Don't resist them; that only creates sorrow. Let reality be reality. Let things flow naturally forward in whatever way they like."**
> **~ Lao Tzu**

Chapter 4

Facing a Harsh Reality

♥

"You have power over your mind, not outside events. Realize this, and you will find strength."
~ Marcus Aurelius

The Scary Aftermath

As I processed my recent diagnosis, many hard and depressing questions flashed relentlessly through my mind:

AMANDA FELIZ

What stage of cancer was it?

Am I going to live?

Am I going to die?

What about my kids?

What about work?

What about rent?

What about food?

What about all the shit in my house?

Who's going to go through all that?

Who's going to take care of my kids?

Will I lose my hair?

Will I need chemo?

Will I need surgery?

Will I be weak?

What am I going to do?

Will I still feel like a woman if my natural breasts are different?

What size was this thing?

Was it taking over my entire body?

How did things get this far?

What now?

Am I going to make the right choices?

Some of these questions led me to become extremely adamant that I needed to continue working. I wanted to avoid my finances spiraling out of control at all costs. I knew that if I did not work, I was not going to have a reliable income and therefore would not be able to cater to all of our vital needs. Most simply, I needed to work because we needed to eat, and we needed rent money to have a roof over our heads. Most critically, if we did not have a place to live, it would be very devastating to be dealing with cancer and homelessness at the same time.

I was really scared, to say the least. One of my biggest fears has always been not being able to provide a stable home for me and my kids. The cost of housing had been rising quickly, outpacing incomes plus education costs, and paying rent was a constant struggle no matter the level of education I had. It felt like any time I improved my learning for a better life, the rate of inflation increased so much. It still is a fear of mine as inflation continues to grow like mad.

Talking to My Kids

Since Angela and Wesley were with me at the DA's office when I received the phone call about my diagnosis, they were well aware that something was going on. They stayed in the waiting room while I met with the DA, and then we all went home to talk. Wes was only nine and too young to comprehend the situation at hand, but Angela was mature enough to understand that something serious was amiss.

On our drive home, they asked me a few times what happened on the phone, and I explained that I would tell them later. Once we got home, I told my kids that it was time for us to sit down and talk. Once we got settled, I let them know that the call I got earlier was not good news: it had been the doctor's office, and I was diagnosed with breast cancer.

In response, they had a lot of questions just like I initially did: what would happen next? would I be okay? was I going to die? would they be able to see me at the hospital? would they be able to stay home?

Most of all, they were a little scared, so we shared a family hug. I did what any good mom would do, reassuring them that everything would be okay. At the same time, in the back of my mind, I was deeply sad and scared for my kids because of my own lingering questions.

In the days to come, I remember telling my kids that it was very important for them to take care of themselves and their health. Before my diagnosis, it was always a mild warning because of the family history of cancer. After my diagnosis, I emphasized the need for them even more so, especially now that their own mother had cancer as well!

Breaking the News to Friends and Family

One of the hardest things I had to do next was to tell my friends and family about my diagnosis.

I started making phone calls to let the closest people in my immediate circles know that I had just been diagnosed with breast cancer.

What an emotionally draining process! Even though I subconsciously held this optimism that I was going to be okay, my message did not convey the same sentiment. Friends and families often responded to the news as if I were already dead, even though I was still very much alive. Of course, I couldn't blame anyone for feeling this way, since most cancers have no cure and those diagnoses are a death sentence most of the time.

Another difficult part of handling these depressive phone calls was that I never knew how each person would react. Each time I told another friend or family member, I lived the pain of finding out about my own cancer and dealing with it again over and over until I didn't have anyone else to tell.

School vacation was still going on at that point, so I was spared from having to talk to all of my coworkers, but I had the chance to confide in several teacher friends whom I worked with and had a bit of a closer relationship with at the time. I was at my mom's house for a sleepover, which really helped me both deal with the news and enjoy something fun. I took the opportunity to express that I was bummed about my diagnosis.

In response, four of us decided to go out and have a drink together to shake off that news a little bit. That really helped me, because it made me realize that regardless of what I was going through, I would have supportive people in my corner.

On my way to meet my friends, I also called up *mi primo hermano*, my first cousin who is like a brother to me. In our Spanish family, five of us first cousins were very close—four boys and me, the only girl. I had a few other cousins, including a girl first cousin, but we weren't close. Two of the four boys were younger than me, so I was like their big sister when we were growing up together. I had always been closest with one in particular, so I called him *mi hermano*.

When I called, my cousin was in high spirits. He had just bought a house, which made my news all the more sad because I had to dampen his mood.

"Hey, guess what!" he greeted me. "I just signed papers on a house!"

"That's awesome!" I replied, "But, guess what? I just found out I have breast cancer!" What a delivery!

My friends were very supportive and empathetic, and they encouraged me to let them know if I needed anything. I came to understand that their words, "Let me know what you need," actually and truly meant, "I want to help you, but I don't know how."

Meanwhile, my aunt was so kind as to pay for a cleaner to come in and help me clean my house a couple of times. What a gift! Plus, it was quite the surprise coming from her in particular, which is a story for another time.

It was very hard to stay positive throughout the whole process of breaking my sad news to everyone, but their reactions were always kind. They didn't want me to die! I learned that my friends and family needed to hear positive, reassuring words just as much as I did. The only challenge was when I suddenly felt as if I had to be positive for THEM! I know this seems so bizarre, but it was the sad truth! They NEEDED me to tell them I was going to be okay and share any little wins with them so that they were reassured that I truly was going to be all right.

Beginning the Treatment Process

Shortly after my diagnosis, my mother and a good friend went with me to the first doctor's appointment. While they were primarily there for emotional support, I also found it helpful to have another set of ears to pay attention to the medical jargon that was being thrown around. It was very comforting and convenient for me to have both of them accompany me because they helped ask the right questions and sought clarifications about the next steps.

In fact, I didn't realize how valuable this support was until I was in the thick of it. My mind was often clouded during the appointments, so I was grateful that someone else could listen to every explanation and hear things that I didn't necessarily hear, might have missed, or interpreted a little differently. I tried to open up, ask questions, and take notes, but there was a lot of information coming my way. I had to answer so many questions and process a lot of details, but often I was unsure about the questions that I needed to ask. So, I was very thankful that I had other people with me for both the emotional and clarity aspects.

> Dear Lord, please give me strength as I travel through this journey of healing. Please guide the doctors and keep me safe. Please watch over my family, my friends and keep them safe. Thank-you
> Amen

My mom's prayer for me during my healing journey

Then there was the medical team to sort out and understand. I felt like I was constantly in motion, going from person to person to person, and had to constantly figure out who each person was, what their role was, what they were asking of me, and how to best answer their questions. Throughout my interactions with the medical staff, I found them to be nice, average people, not extra sweet but straightforward when telling me what I needed to do.

The oncology doctors, the surgeon, the on-call nurses, and the other medical staff often invited me to ask them any questions about any details I didn't understand. Each one did their best to be helpful and explain what their role was when I first met them. I even had a team of nurses talk to me and provide me with pamphlets so that I could better understand what was happening in each step of the procedures. Still, there were so many people and details to keep track of!

The appointments were frequent at the beginning as everyone prepped me for treatment. The doctors and their medical staff did their best to inform me about the treatment process and the desired or expected prognosis, based on the treatment of other patients with similar diagnoses. They provided me with all the information I needed to know about each phase of treatment and what was involved, although it did not allay my fears and anxiety about the knowns and unknowns.

Despite the staff's meticulous attention to every bit of information, sometimes little details fell through the cracks. For instance, before my first treatment was scheduled, I got a phone call to verify that I was getting my IUD removed. I had a hormone-based cancer, so I would need to have that taken out before any treatments could take place. This took me by surprise, and now I had to call in for a time to have that removed.

So, I was left with a big question: "How could such an important detail fall through the cracks?" Even now, it still baffles me! Such an oversight could have delayed the start of my treatments.

As I prepared for the next step, I was anxious about chemotherapy and its effect on my life. I knew that it was inevitable that I was going to lose my hair, which would consequently assault my sense of beauty and self-esteem. Yet, if chemo saved my life, I knew that I would live to grow hair another day, or so I hoped! Things could not get much worse, right? And yet, I constantly wondered, "I am a hair twirler, so what about my twirl?'

Financial Difficulty

During this time of preparing for the start of treatments, my main focus was to address how my economic stability could be severely affected by receiving chemo. After all, I was a single mother of two and the sole breadwinner of our family. Like, seriously, what do single moms do when faced with this same situation if they can not work?

I didn't even have enough time to try to figure these questions out! I needed energy to heal, and I needed to keep working during the treatment process. At the time, I was working paycheck to paycheck, so my finances were not enough to allow me to stay out of work during my treatment. And, of course, I had no savings. If I had savings, perhaps my finances would not have consumed so much of my time and thoughts.

I was extremely anxious that my ability to continue working was going to be affected, and I had many sleepless nights over it. I just *had* to work, but I did not know how I was going to be able to work while facing the expectedly unexpected side effects of cancer treatments. I didn't know if I'd get just one side effect, or some, or all of them! So, I continued to keep worrying about how my bills were going to get paid and how I was going to feed and clothe my children during the upcoming ordeal.

At a minimum, we just needed a roof over our heads. Yet, paying rent without an income was scary. To me, it seemed like a terrifying cycle: if I couldn't work because of cancer, then I wouldn't be able to pay rent, and if I couldn't pay rent, would I now end up homeless because of cancer??? The looming rent issue made me feel like every time I took a tiny step forward, I ended up landing two steps back. Then there was the other big issue: I not only needed the money, but I didn't want to sit at home to heal and face thoughts that would have me dead!

To relieve some of my stress, I told myself that I was determined to keep working unless the doctors told me differently. I was going to push myself to continue working until I was physically unable to. Looking back, I believe a lot of that hard work and determination is what helped keep me alive. Work distracted me from constantly being preoccupied with sorrowful and depressing thoughts. With each passing moment, I did not want to tread into deeper darkness by crafting a sad story where I was imagining what life could have been, things I had not done and now wished I could do, or why this was happening to me. I even avoided thoughts of what would happen if treatments did not work. I had to survive for my kids, so I kept fighting!

At the same time, I held another secret worry about what would happen if I were to die. After my divorce, I had moved from a large three-bedroom house with an office to a very small two-bedroom house without an office, requiring me to get rid of some stuff. I thought that the new move would be temporary, so I stored a lot of things in the basement. After I started teaching, however, I began collecting anything and everything that was free so I wouldn't have to go out and buy all the stuff I needed as a classroom teacher.

My house had suddenly become a hoarder's house! So, when I harbored thoughts that I might die, I immediately felt bad for the person who would have to do the clean-up. I decided that if I was going to die, I had to organize and clean up the house before that happened. I eventually did start to clean it up, too, which was a slow process that took several years and is still ongoing in different ways.

In retrospect, it's a scary situation to be in when you are constantly worried, whether about your living situation, your accumulated belongings, or even your own funeral! While your mind can take you to exhilarating places where you win the lottery and live your happiest life ever, it can also take you in the opposite direction where dark thoughts, depression, and sorrow dwell.

I constantly expressed my biggest worry to my doctor about whether I was going to be able to work or not. He did not have a definite answer for me at that time, saying that he would have to wait until the treatment began, as he could not predict how I was going to tolerate chemotherapy both physically and mentally. His best answer for me was that everything depended on how my body reacted. He told me I could continue to work for now, but we would revisit my working at a later date.

Despite that positive answer, I kept asking the doctor if I was going to be able to work, insisting that I *needed* to be able to work. Throughout it all, my mother lovingly continued to tell me to stop worrying about work because I did not need to be stressing those details when my greatest concern at that moment should be my health. Unfortunately, her reminders did not stop me from worrying about where I was going to live, what I was going to eat, where I was going to sleep, and how I would provide for my children's well-being—all in the event that I was unable to work. This was my sad reality, and I never told anyone the deep truth about why I was so adamant about working.

One thing was for sure: I couldn't have my kids going through any hard times, and thus, I could not afford the burden of not working in addition to going through treatments! I even thought, "Okay, cancer, I got this. I'm going to beat you!" In hindsight, I truly think that if I had been consumed by negative thoughts, it would have taken over me, and I would have been done.

As many times as I mention that I was afraid of not being able to pay rent, I want to emphasize that it is a very real and important concern that is not properly addressed in America. I'm sure that many others like me have struggled with the whole housing concern, feeling a little bit of relief when you get just one foot ahead to pay for rent comfortably. But then, rent goes up, leaving you with the necessity to go back to school, face school debt, and try to get ahead in the employment realm so you can pay for housing expenses, which will only continue to increase. It is a crazy cycle!

So, what can be done about it? This is a real and serious question to ask anyone who is facing cancer. While everything else is taken care of for cancer patients, housing is just not one of those things. Without housing, it is just adding stress, and this at a time when you need to try and be as stress-free as possible. Having cancer treatments and being highly stressed is counterproductive to your health! As I have often wondered, since insurance should help with anything to alleviate any stress during cancer, why can't these companies cover the loss of a job or regular income so parents facing cancer treatments are able to go home and hug their kids?

Even as I struggled during this time with many worries and anxiety, I was determined to stay positive. As the saying goes, when life hands you a lemon, you must try and make lemonade. Also, misery loves company, so the more miserable and sad you are, the more you will feel that way. Instead, I always tried to find a silver lining in the dark clouds. I told myself constantly, "Try to be positive! No matter how hard it is!" After all, there is always a glimmer of hope, no matter how hopeless we think a situation is.

Teaching with Cancer

Meanwhile, as the school year approached, I was thinking about the further education classes I needed to take to further my career in teaching and really be able to continue teaching. I had already passed the MTELs, which were broken down according to subject matter, and I wanted to focus on teaching elementary grades as an English learning teacher.

So, I began focusing on the education I needed for that category. The requirement was that I complete a master's in teaching within five years of beginning to teach with my preliminary teacher's license, so the pressure was on! I calculated that I would need one year for breast cancer treatments and one year for recovery, so here was even more stress!

The hardest part to face was that my progress in the teaching world was very exciting, but I felt like I had just been given a severe punch in my gut. How was I going to keep my career and be excited about obtaining my master's while a personal catastrophe was going on?

Ever optimistic, I was determined to press on by prioritizing my health while finding a program that would work for my schedule. Fortunately, I discovered a year-long program called Class Measures that cost about $2500, which was a back-door resolution for anyone who couldn't get their master's in the allotted time. As a state-approved option, I found a little hope in that!

Now, my next step was to determine where I would get the money for Class Measures! Once again, I was facing another situation on top of everything else that caused me stress and anxiety. The only way I was able to deal with all the crushing pressures of life at that time was by taking each thing as it came at that moment. I often made a list of the day-to-day tasks to give me focus for each step that was right in front of me.

After much worrying, I finally got the news that I had practically begged for, which was my primary drive at the moment: I could continue working through my cancer treatments! The doctor told me that since it was toward the end of flu season, I would be able to continue working at school. His only requirement was that I remember to keep the windows open as much as possible and wash my hands frequently. It was a go! What a huge, major relief! No added housing stress!

Once I got this exciting news, I began to think about what to tell my students. I knew that chemo would make me lose my hair, so I wanted to tell the students in my classroom about the visible changes they were going to see in me ahead of time. I planned a day to break the news and also brought in the school's social worker who let the kids know she was available in case any of them needed to talk.

With that, I told my students how I was sick, would be receiving treatment, and that they would see physical changes in me, most notably the loss of my hair. The kids all stared at me with blank faces as they tried their best to understand, asking if I would still be their teacher. I assured them that I would be there as much as I could be, and that we would all keep the windows open and wash our hands, just to reiterate what the doctors told me. I told my students that if we all did this together, then I had a high chance of being at school with them every day.

My Wonderful Network of Support

All throughout this time, I had a great support system in place thanks to my teacher friends. For example, my friends and acquaintances helped a great deal in looking out for Wesley, who had been active in baseball for the past five years, whether that meant dropping him off, picking him up, or just keeping an eye on him while I was at work.

One of my coworkers initiated a meal plan, and the rest of my coworkers signed up to create a whole meal system for me, which I greatly appreciated! My teacher friends would bring the meals to school if they knew I was going to be at work that day, or they would even drop them off at my doorstep at home. To make the process even easier, they had a whole website where people signed up and listed what they were going to bring!

The meal plan was so helpful in providing my kids with dinner every night, taking the guesswork out of mealtime, and even providing leftovers for the next day. Even when I couldn't eat a whole lot, it was so nice to have healthier meals on the table. I was especially happy to give this food to my kids and watch them enjoy it!

My colleagues at work also organized a paint party for me where we created a work of art while enjoying drinks and snacks. They collected money and gave me donations to help out with the associated costs of the treatment journey. It was such a wonderful time and also very emotional to see how everyone was coming together to support me financially and show their love.

Another day, my school held a dress-down day for me where everyone got to wear jeans and donate whatever they wished to show their support and love to keep me going. I still have all their thoughtful cards with beautiful messages! The donations given to me were a huge help for meals, medicines, and more. My second-grade team of teachers also got matching t-shirts for us all to wear. Not only was I surprised by this, but I was so happy they thought of the idea!

To this day, I really appreciate all of the gestures of kindness bestowed upon me by my colleagues. All their acts of help and support brought me so much relief both emotionally and physically from the burden of juggling everything that needed to be done on my own.

Out of all of those touching moments, I will always remember the day when I went to work after having an awful night and struggling through the next morning. It was one of the worst days of all, since I hadn't felt so yucky before now, but this day took the prize.

After arriving at school, I struggled to keep my composure as I headed down the halls to my classroom door. As I opened my door, I saw something completely unexpected. There, on my desk, was the most beautiful single yellow flower.

I was suddenly overwhelmed with immense joy! It was as if a ray of hope had burst upon me with a message that said, "It will all be okay!" Just a few moments ago, I was feeling so terrible, but that had all been washed away. I was so happy that I had been able to push myself to go to school. Someone else had been there before me, bringing in the sun to brighten up my whole day! I shed happy tears of joy after that and was immediately at peace, reminded that I had a team behind me to help when things got really tough.

"Many people will walk in and out of your life, but only true friends will leave footprints in your heart."
~ Eleanor Roosevelt

Chapter 5

My Treatment Journey

♥

> "Life is a journey that must be traveled no matter how bad the roads and accommodations."
> ~ Oliver Goldsmith

My Timeline

In reflecting on my treatment journey and my victory over cancer, this is the timeline of events that I faced:

August 2013: I discovered the lump in my left breast.

December 2013: I experienced repeated lingering colds and constipation for the first time ever.

February 2014: I received a cancer diagnosis.

April 2014: I started chemotherapy treatments.

June 2024: I successfully completed chemotherapy.

July 2014: I enjoyed a month of rest and recovery before surgery.

August 2014: I underwent surgery to remove the cancer, followed by another period of recovery.

October 2014: I began radiation treatment.

November 2014: I rang the bell to signify that the period of cancer treatment was over!

To Lumpectomy or to Mastectomy—That is the Question!

The opening line of Hamlet's soliloquy, "To be, or not to be," discusses the theme of existential crisis, which succinctly describes the predicament I was facing shortly after my diagnosis. My doctor's office first called me to schedule various appointments with specialists. So, shortly afterward, on one morning at the end of February, I met with three doctors to go over the details of my treatment.

Of the three doctors, one was the Medical Oncologist, one was the Radiation Oncologist, and the last was a General Practitioner. They each provided me with reading material that would be a helpful reference in the days ahead. They also explained that my order of treatment would begin with chemotherapy to reduce the tumor, which was about 4.5 centimeters in size. After that, if the tumor responded well to the chemo and decreased in size, I would undergo surgery to remove the reduced tumor. Finally, I would undergo radiation that would kill the cancer cells and slow down their future growth by damaging their DNA, since cancer cells whose DNA is damaged beyond repair stop dividing and die (see Resources page for more details).

At that point, I had a decision to make: would I choose a lumpectomy or a mastectomy? The doctors told me to make an appointment with a plastic surgeon to discuss the surgical options. It was a difficult choice to make! Which of the two was the best for me? Should I have one whole breast removed or just have the lump removed? If I had the breast removed, what about my other breast? The thought of missing a breast was hard enough to comprehend and accept!

Yet, if I had one breast removed, I also had the option of having them both removed.

When I first began to learn about all the medical details related to cancer, I felt overwhelmed. A lot of stuff was going on! I had a lot of quick decisions to make that were mixed up along with a lot of new medical jargon. I felt that if I had time to figure these things out or research them, it would be easier, but there was no time. My head was spinning! I desperately hoped that I was making the right decision in each case. I knew that it wouldn't be until much later when I was feeling better that I would be able to reflect and look back, saying that I either made the right decision or not. Yet, at that point, I would be left with my decision and wouldn't be able to reverse it anyway. *¡La vida es asi!*

Plastic Surgeon Appointment

My next stop was to see a plastic surgeon. My mother accompanied me to my appointment at MGH, and it was an absolutely awful experience. To start off, the doctor was so f-ing rude! I literally wanted to punch him in the face! He left a sore taste in my mouth, I never wanted to hear his name again, and I would never ever recommend him.

Because I was chubbier at the time, he started out within minutes of his examination by looking at me and saying matter-of-factly, "I thought your boobs would be a lot bigger in proportion to your body." He was implying that I was fat with little breasts! Even though he tried to express his view in nice medical terms, he could not hide his tinge of sarcasm. He was arrogant, did not have bedside manners, and did not care about me. At the end of the day, he would get his paycheck regardless of his attitude. I was just a number that was referred to him! I didn't care how true this information might have been; he was tacky!

Then, when I asked him a question about the procedure, he answered my question in medical jargon. I looked at him in disbelief because my mother was with me, so I asked him if he could say that again in layman's terms. Instead, he just repeated himself in the same exact way, except that he used an arrogant tone and simply spoke slower, as if I was dumb and my mother was dumber.

I looked at him again and said, "I understood you when you said it the first time, but that's not how I asked you to say it." It was my way of giving a bit of attitude back!

After we walked out of his office, I looked at my mother and said to her, "There's no chance in hell that I would ever allow myself to be put asleep, completely unconscious, and have him do what over my body?! Big nope!"

So, I ruled that doctor out immediately and continued my search to find another plastic surgeon. Fortunately, I successfully found another specialist and scheduled yet another appointment for a future date.

Genetic Testing

In February, I went through many tests, including the breast cancer (BRCA) gene test to check for my risk of breast and ovarian cancer (see the Resources for more details). As I learned, this was necessary to see if I inherited harmful variants or mutations that could be passed on to my daughter. Depending on the results, Angela might need to be careful earlier on in her young womanhood and be closely monitored for any developing signs of cancer.

Fortunately, my test results showed that the cancer was not hereditary, which was a relief for my daughter's sake! Basically, my situation in getting breast cancer was just my usual case of woes in life.

Relieved by that news, I went on to face other tests: a CAT scan, an injection, and a bone test. Every time I underwent more procedures, I always had to wait for the results and see how they would affect my overall treatment.

Making a Decision

In March, it was time for my appointment with a different plastic surgeon. I vividly remember how the office was set up like a beautiful spa environment with lovely minimalist decorations like little sculpted waterfalls. As soon as I walked in, I felt the peaceful aura, as if by simply entering, all my troubles would melt away. I remember thinking that I loved the space because of its alluring Zen decorations and calming environment, and how I would love to replicate that calming environment for my own home!

As part of the procedural requirements of having me as a patient, the staff had to take before-and-after pictures. The plastic surgeon and his assistant took pictures of my top half from both the back and the front. As I learned, plastic surgery is usually an elective surgery for cosmetic purposes, but on rare occasions, it is used for breast reconstruction after a lumpectomy or mastectomy. It is also a lucrative business for plastic surgeons, so they really tried to persuade me to have a whole mastectomy so I would receive new reconstructed breasts.

I listened carefully as they promised to fix my whole figure. They told me through the use of illustrations what parts they would remove, the areas they would reconstruct, and the fats they would get rid of. It was an enticing presentation, to say the least!

When I walked out of the plastic surgeon's office, a thought ran through my mind, "Let me find out I got breast cancer and the treatment process might give me a whole freaking new body, the slim one I always wanted with no extra effort! And I don't even have to work for it?" It was a very convincing argument, especially because it would be "medically necessary" following cancer treatment.

Then I decided to do a little digging in an effort to gain an in-depth understanding of the physiology of breast cancer, available treatment options, and what each entailed.

I began researching breast-conserving surgery (lumpectomy) and breast-removal surgery (mastectomy) in great detail, mulling over certain questions to try and make my decision easier:

Was I interested in keeping my breasts? If so, then a lumpectomy followed by radiation might be my best choice.

Did I need my breasts to be as similar in size as possible? A lumpectomy might be better for my appearance, while in rare circumstances, a lumpectomy could make the breast appear smaller or distorted after a greater amount of tissue has been removed.

How worried was I about getting breast cancer again? Mastectomy was an option to consider if removing the entire breast would lessen my anxiety about the possibility of recurrence.

Next, I contemplated plastic surgery and the prospect of getting new boobies and even a new body. Although it was very enticing, if for no other reason other than sexual appeal, there was a lot involved during the post-surgery period. Specifically, I would have to deal with all the surgical drains inserted into the soft tissue of the breast to aid in healing by draining fluid buildup in the area where the breast was removed. If not drained appropriately, excess fluid could cause infections and other complications. The thought of draining and other details did not appeal to me! As a matter of fact, it pushed me away from that idea.

At my latest office visit, I was introduced to another doctor who was one of the best in her field and possibly would be the one to perform my surgery. I called her office and scheduled an appointment with her for later that month. During this next consultation, I was extremely impressed by her honest discussion with me about breast cancer, the surgical options, and the expected outcomes. She simplified medical terms and spoke in layman's terms so I could fully understand what she was explaining to me. This doctor was honest, real, and down-to-earth. She was also blunt, but in a graceful manner.

I remember looking at her and asking, "If you were in my position, what would you do?"

She answered in a very straightforward manner that she would just have the lumpectomy. She proceeded to tell me that a lot of women came to her, thinking that they were going to get a beautiful new body when they had their breasts removed and reconstructed. However, she explained that most women think that the flap under the arm is removed with the breast, but in actuality, that is side fat and is not removed.

From there, she began to talk about how each person's perception of themselves will change. Specifically after a mastectomy, the perception changes because, as a woman, you're not going to be comfortable having a flat chest like a boy. Once again, she reminded me about the side fat, and then we also discussed the recovery process for each type of procedure.

After having such an in-depth discussion with this doctor, I was convinced to just have the lump removed. My research helped confirm this decision, since it was not so cosmetically involved and would not be taxing on my day-to-day life in the same way that a mastectomy would.

I was already scared of any medical risks, so I wanted to avoid any possible complications from occurring with such an invasive surgery. I already had enough shit happening! Besides that, I was facing a health issue, not an aesthetic issue! When it came down to it, my health was more important than how aesthetically pleasing I would appear following the plastic surgery. No matter how good it sounded to have a whole new body, my main focus was to get better, not go through another complicated ordeal.

More importantly, if I went the mastectomy route, I would need extra care that I definitely didn't want to impose on anyone. I already thought that others might be tired of helping me out, and I didn't want to bother them further! Plus, the thought of trying to recover with someone else helping me with bathroom needs, showering, and other personal things was a lot of added stress for me and for anyone who enlisted to help me. Even to this day, I never want to feel like I'm a burden to anyone!

"I have a lump, and the lump needs to be removed. I don't need the whole boob gone!" I told myself. So, a lumpectomy it was. The entire decision process was stressful, but I was relieved to have come to the right choice, or so I hoped. Besides, with my history, the mastectomy could easily turn into a bigger ordeal than it should be!

As I look back on those days, I realize how hard it is for any cancer patient. Time is short and decisions must be made hard and fast, all because you are required to make a decision quickly.

While I was off doing all of that medical stuff, my home life was in shambles. I was starting chemo, working on the surgery plan, juggling work as a new teacher, helping Wes with baseball, and trying to keep in touch with Angela, who recently decided not to live with us anymore. I constantly worried about my daughter and the hard decisions that I had to make. Plus, I was thinking about Angela's case, which was temporarily paused, but one that we would have to eventually go back to and face.

Angela and I already had a lot of mother-daughter quarrels prior to my diagnosis. My situation added stress to our already stressful house, so Angela came to me at one point and told me that, since she didn't want me to be stressed during my treatments, she was going to move out. And just like that, she was gone, leaving Wes and me to fend for ourselves. I was devastated! I felt like my big baby turned her back on me when I needed her the most.

In response, I tried to make it seem like I was fine as much as I could for Wesley. I took him to his first Red Sox game and Legoland, we went bowling and played billiards, we chilled in the summer when we didn't have work or school, and we got free tickets to Shrek the performance from the 2ShowWeCare organization that helps cancer patients have fun for free. Overall, I tried to give my son as much normal living as possible, or as much normal as living can be!

Like anyone who has ever gone through such hard times, all I could do was just hope that I could sleep at night. It was a vicious cycle of stress! And stress is always that thing keeping you awake at night, even though you are physically exhausted and longing for sleep more than anything. It creeps into your mind, sometimes jolting you out of rest, and makes good rest very difficult.

Chemotherapy Treatments

Shortly after I made the decision about having the lumpectomy, I had an MRI done. From there, I met with a medical oncologist to discuss the plan of events, including the dates and procedures. By the end of the month, I had a port placement done at Union Hospital.

As I soon learned, a port is a device used to draw blood and give treatments, including intravenous fluids, blood transfusions, and drugs like chemotherapy and antibiotics (see the Resources for a sample picture and more information). While I was hesitant to get the port in the first place, I soon recognized its great importance for my upcoming chemo treatments and got it anyway. If I received chemo through an IV each time, it would take three to four hours for a single treatment, and the needle would have to stay in my vein the entire time. If the needle accidentally became displaced at any point, the solution would burn me. The port was not only a safer option, but I would also be able to use my hands while the treatment was taking place and not be restricted.

In early April, I had my very first chemotherapy treatment. After that, I received more chemo every other week on Wednesdays, for a total of eight doses. I had two different kinds of chemotherapy medicines, one for the first four treatments and the other for the remaining four treatments. The scary part of one of those medicines, which was Doxorubicin or Adriamycin, was that I was told that I could only have so much of that in my entire lifetime because of the damage it does to your cardiac muscle tissue. The medical staff told me this as something I needed to remember just in case something came up so I could say that I already had my full share.

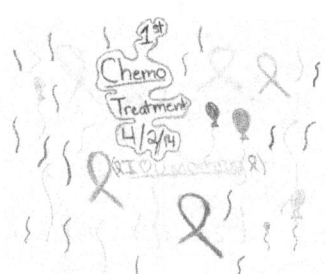

Wesley's beautiful picture for my first treatment

Around this time, Wesley was playing baseball, which was a relief to me because he was always away from me during those vulnerable moments when I was suffering from the chemotherapy after-effects. I did not want him to see me like that! His tenth birthday was coming up, and he happened to have a game, so some of the other parents and I decided to celebrate with a cake down at the field with some of Wes's friends after the game ended. I clearly remember that time because I was beginning to lose my hair and wondered if I was going to wear a wig.

Before each chemotherapy dose, the medical staff drew some of my blood for laboratory analysis to ascertain if I would be able to withstand the treatment that day. This took about an hour or an hour and a half, while the treatment itself was three to four hours.

When I learned about the value of blood count and could access the preliminary report on the online patient portal, I started looking up the details online as a self-assessment tool to check for any abnormalities. Unfortunately, my Google results would always show me that I was close to being dead!

As a result, I would quickly become all panicky and freaked out, but then I would soon get a call from the doctor saying that the results from the lab said that I was perfectly fine. When the medical staff learned that I was looking up my blood count online, they told me not to because the internet diagnosis would freak me out, but I kept doing it quite often!

Eventually, after enough poking and pricking, I developed a rash in the area where tape was used after blood was drawn. My skin was irritated, and that was a new issue to deal with.

After each chemotherapy treatment, I walked out of the hospital feeling okay. The next day, I felt so energetic, like a powerhouse! My mother noticed how much energy I had and would always be fascinated by what they were giving me to make me so energized. I felt like Superwoman! I could build Rome in a day! I never had so much energy in my life! It was an almost amazing feeling to feel superhuman, like I could conquer everything and get so much done at a fast speed.

This period of having so much energy and feeling amazing, unfortunately, was short-lived.

I quickly learned to make sure things around the house were in order on those powerhouse days so when I crashed and burned I wouldn't feel overwhelmed. Some time from mid-morning to early afternoon the day after my super energy day, my energy levels and motivation would deteriorate rapidly and stay like that for the rest of the week and through the weekend. I often ended up missing work on Mondays and sometimes on Tuesdays, finally regaining my basic energy levels on Wednesdays. I then was able to finish my work week, as I was determined to continue working all throughout my treatment period. Then the following week would come, and the treatment and roller-coaster energy cycle would continue all over again—sixteen long weeks in a row.

The After-Effects of Chemo

For each chemotherapy treatment, I set aside three to four hours to sit in place at the hospital for the two different kinds of medicine to be injected into my body. After the first few treatments, I received a self-inflicting drug called Neulasta to boost my immune system at my house, ready to be used the day after my treatment. I hated needles, so self-administering the Neulasta was painful, and I dreaded having to do that every time. However, all throughout the process of fluctuating energy levels and losing my hair, I was stubborn and optimistic, determined to do what I needed to conquer cancer.

I also got a ton of prescriptions to help with all the effects of the chemo like nausea, pain, acid reflux, and more. In reality, it was all stuff to try and tame the poison being put into my body. I already had to deal with enough, so the day I found out that I was paying $40 for an acid reflux prescription that CVS sold over the counter for a lot cheaper, something that the pharmacist never bothered to tell me, was the day I knew the drug industry was horrendous and a bunch of scammers!

Despite the brief moments of feeling like I had super energy, the chemo more often than not gave me a sick and achy internal feeling down to my bones. I was eager to be healthy again! *¡Por el amor a Dios!*

After the eight chemo treatments were finally over, I so badly wanted the medical port still attached to my chest to be removed. So, when talking to the medical staff after the last chemo was over, my first question was, "Can I get the port taken out?"

The doctor and team, unfortunately, were slow to give me a straight answer. After I pressed multiple times, I finally got a reply, "Well, technically, yes, but we recommend that it stay in, just in case anything happens."

In my mind, I was loudly protesting. "What could possibly happen? Treatments were done! Get this thing out of me!"

I was tired of being poked and pricked, and this was even before the surgery and radiation. I couldn't think of anything negative happening as a result of taking the port out, so I kept pressing. Finally, I got my desired result, and the medical team agreed and took the port out. What a relief!

That night, I got very sick. I was sweating, my stomach hurt very badly, and I was trying to pee, but I couldn't. The pain made me want to throw up, but I couldn't do that either.

After being in so much pain all night long, I waited until the crack of dawn to call my mom. I told her that I had been sick for many hours and felt like I needed to go to the emergency room. Mom came to my rescue and took me to Union Hospital, which is where I not only had my port put in but also had it removed.

As the medical staff began to ask me what happened, I explained my symptoms. In the back of my mind, I was filled with dread. "It's because I made them take out the port when I was advised to wait a little bit!" I thought to myself.

Since I still felt so nauseous, the staff gave me something to get rid of the nausea. I felt better and was finally able to relax and get comfortable. I lay in the hospital bed, not even moving and full of relief. After some time, I still felt better, so the staff told me they were preparing to discharge me.

Meanwhile, my mom was saying, "You didn't even do any tests, all you did was give her anti-nausea medicine!"

As soon as the staff told me that they were going to discharge me, however, the pain started up all over again. No one was sure what was happening, but then my mom came to the rescue once again and suggested that they check me for kidney stones. She told the nurse that my symptoms matched what happened when she was trying to pass them. The nurse looked at my mom as if mesmerized!

After running some tests and checking me over, the hospital staff found that I had not just one or two but multiple kidney stones! As if that wasn't enough, one of the stones was so big that they had to do surgery and use a stent to get it out!

This was not the first time that my body reacted negatively to the chemotherapy by developing kidney stones. On two other occasions, the medical staff had to use shock waves to break up the stones inside of me before they could be safely passed.

What a horrible experience! On top of the cancer treatments that I had dealt with, this was a whole new ordeal to contend with! I had to see a urologist on a regular basis for a little while and get a 24-hour analysis done every so often to prevent the kidney stones from continuing to occur.

One day, I was getting ready to leave for one of my appointments with the urologist, and there was a sudden knock on my door. I wondered who that could be, since I had just moved there and nobody knew I lived there yet. Well, it was some man from the Isabella Stewart Gardner

Museum at my door, telling me something so bizarre that I thought my safety was at risk and had to wait for him to leave. Meanwhile, I was stressed about getting to my appointment on time.

Those appointments went on for a while until I discovered one of the best-kept secrets to preventing the buildup of kidney stones in the first place: drinking plenty of water with freshly-squeezed lemon in it. As painful as all of that was to go through, I was relieved that it had nothing to do with removing the port but was definitely another one of the effects of chemo.

Through all of my treatments, I was very thankful for the support and positivity. As easy as it is to feel like you are alone in these aspects, you really are not alone. Every time I was out sick with chemo treatments, especially on the third day following treatments and through the end of that week, I had to be prepared by leaving plans for my sub for a couple of days. Sometimes it was especially difficult since I was still a very new teacher, learning the new ropes and trying to juggle everything.

In the end, I was very thankful most of all that I was able to work! I was willing to take any extra steps just to feel secure that I would not face a housing issue on top of everything else. Plus, I believe that focusing on work helped me get through everything. Your mind can go crazy and get stuck in a rabbit hole if you don't have something to do while dealing with cancer or anything else that might be detrimental to your well-being. So, I was very grateful to be able to stay busy, keep my mind occupied, and not constantly obsess about everything else that was happening.

Surgery and Radiation

After my chemo was over, the doctors allowed time for my immune system to build back up so that I could safely tolerate surgery and any complications that might have arisen from it. They had me wait about a month after my last chemo and then did the surgery.

This ordeal was a same-day procedure of having the lump removed and a few lymph nodes for testing, so the doctors simply gave me post-surgery instructions and sent me home. As I recovered from that surgery, I was told to wait another month or so before radiation was to begin. The reason for the recovery period was for the scar tissue to heal before it received the radiation therapy.

After the surgery and my second time of rest was behind me, I faced the next ordeal: radiation. As a first step, I received four little tattoos in the form of dots in a certain area to mark where the radiation machine would line up every time.

Those little tattooed dots were permanent, and it was kind of a joke because I had never gotten any other tattoos before then. Yet, deep down inside, it was also hard to acknowledge that the reason for my first tattoos was because of cancer! I had heard of cancer survivors who got pretty tattoos afterward to cover up the dots, with the point of making an elaborate tattoo to celebrate their victory. I thought about doing that also, but here was another sad part about the whole situation: the doctors recommended that even if the dots were covered up, they should still always remain somewhat visible in case they needed to be used again in the future! *¿En serio?*

The radiation process meant going in every day, Monday through Friday, for a total of

33 treatments. Each time, I went to a specific location in the hospital, got undressed, had a machine hone in on the specific area on my body, and had the radiation done. Everything was over within an hour, but it became externally draining to have to go for a treatment every day of the week. After a couple of weeks, the whole area became extremely dry and a nuisance, so I remember my son helping me put tons of lotion on my skin in an effort to soften it up.

In total, my radiation treatment translated into a little over six weeks. Meanwhile, it was October, so I was trying to balance the rest of my life while devoting time each day for treatment. I was a new teacher at the school, Wes was in regular school plus fall ball practice, and Angela had already moved out to try and alleviate any tension between us, which only served to worry me even more!

On top of that, since it was October, the traffic was crazy when driving from my town of Lynn through Salem to get to MGH in Danvers. If you know anything about Salem, MA, then you know it is very busy in October because of the increased tourism around Halloween. When the new school year started, the original plan was to have me go to MGH at 4:00 or 5:00 PM, which meant going through Salem at a time when people were just getting out of work and traffic was significantly heavier. To make matters worse, I was getting home extremely late because of this as well. It was like a mini horror show to drive through SALEM traffic to and from MGH every day in OCTOBER. Like, "Ha, the joke is on you!"

In fact, one of the first radiation treatments had me so stressed out because of the time and traffic being so heavy that the doctors had a discussion with me. They told me that they couldn't do the treatment on me when I was so stressed out, so we worked out a solution. I began going for radiation after school got out, when traffic didn't have a chance to pick up and was not as crazy.

This plan worked better. Each day, I would either drop Wes off at baseball practice or he would accompany me to radiation. When Wes came with me, we would listen to tunes on the way up to MGH. When he had baseball practice, I had friends bring Wes home afterward so I could go straight home and relax. Most of the time, it was his coaches who dropped him off, and it reminded me of how influential and beneficial baseball has always been in my son's life. I was so grateful for not only the help but for the true distraction it served him.

I didn't always go straight home and relax after I finished radiation. Sometimes, I returned to school to do lesson plans for two or three hours before heading home. I would text the custodian if I had to go back and work, and he would very kindly let me back into the building since my badge didn't work after hours. I was always grateful that he was available to let me in so I could be prepared to teach the next day. The custodian and I sometimes dreamed of winning the lottery so we didn't have to work, and we joked that we would split it. To this day, I still think about that. If I won the lottery now, I would still give him a cut!

After the month-and-a-half-long radiation ordeal was over, there were other permanent things to deal with. The biggest factor was extremely dry skin that needed to be slathered up with lotion as many times a day as possible. It took months of lotion for the area to be healed, and to this day, I still feel a bit of numbing sensation in that radiation area.

Then, from the lumpectomy surgery, I had an incision made beneath my armpit, so I have a lasting scar there. The doctors also checked the lymph nodes for any sign of cancer and said that while there was still a little bit left, we cleared the margins enough so that it was no longer a big threat.

Always Staying Positive

While my whole treatment journey was difficult, the thing that kept me going was that I was able to work. This was a huge benefit both financially and emotionally. When you're willing to do whatever it takes to keep your mind busy, you keep yourself from things getting worse. The alternative for me was looking things up online, creating scary scenarios in my mind, and putting myself in a negative space to deal with this catastrophic illness that can become even more tragic. By keeping my mind busy and knowing that I could still do things, it helped me know that things were going to be okay instead of driving myself mad with thoughts about death.

About a month into my prognosis, the principal at the school I was working at shared with me in confidence that her sister-in-law had also been diagnosed with breast cancer. However, she confided in me that her sister-in-law was not taking the situation in hand the way I did, according to her observation. The principal was alluding to the fact that I still came to work every day and tried to be happy and jolly so that I could get done what needed to be accomplished, even when I might not have felt like it.

So, the principal asked me for my opinion or any advice because her sister-in-law was so miserable by deciding to just sit at home and feel bad for herself. I responded by telling her that it is understandable to be depressed and miserable about a cancer diagnosis, but that it is more beneficial to not have a pity party for yourself and to try to keep doing things that you were doing before. I told her that I found it helpful to keep my mind occupied with positive things and finding light in the day-to-day.

I say the same thing to anyone who might struggle with a cancer diagnosis and their own resulting treatment journey: find something to focus on, even if it's just one little thing. Pick up a little hobby or something to look forward to every day that makes you happy. Read a book or otherwise keep your mind busy so you think about positive things instead of filling your mind with negativity. Then, when you are thinking negatively, remember that it's a fast and serious hole that you can easily fall into. It's much better to go for a small walk, call a friend, write, read, watch a movie, or so many other things. I know it is easier said than done, but that rabbit hole can be pretty disastrous.

Thinking over my whole treatment journey, so many small memories come back to me about how hard it was. I faced so many unpleasant things during the treatments: PET scans, drinking that awful chalky drink, not being able to pee for a certain amount of time, getting jabbed with needles, having to stab myself with needles also, and so many other things you don't want to do. One time, I remember that the treatment caused me to be in so much physical pain that I almost yelled out, all while trying to hold it back from Wes because he was witnessing it. Thinking back, all of these are very sensitive topics because the chemotherapy treatments really took a toll on me.

On a positive note, however, for as many difficult things that happened, there were many special things as well. On days when I was out of energy, my teacher colleagues stepped in to help out. They set up that wonderful meal-sharing plan to bring me a meal once a week. The meal sharing became especially handy on my chemo days, so I did not have to worry about cooking food for the next couple of days.

My colleagues also surprised me with cards, notes, thoughts, and tokens. The notes were especially helpful on down days! The fact that they were thinking of me was more than I could imagine, and it was a very big deal to me. The endless cards and thoughtful gestures really carried me through, and I really appreciate the teachers and their efforts. It was extraordinarily nice of them to help me!

Another big thing for me was not having to worry about waiting for Wesley when he was in baseball for a game or practice. When a friend or coach brought him home so I could rest, that was truly PRICELESS!!!

While I didn't even know if I was going to have a team fighting for me during my treatment journey, my angels put a strong team in my corner that carried me through. You see, while I was dealing with all of this, I wondered if it was going to kill me. I wondered if this would be the end or if there was something more. I had heard of so many crazy stories of accidents: things like tires flying across the other side of the highway, trees falling, sinking holes in the ground, and more. All of these things ended up killing people, and I am still here!

I even had a dear high school acquaintance who was my age and had a different kind of cancer. She and I had our battles around the same time. We would message each other for support and see how the chemo treatments were going.

She had a child who was younger than Wes, and her treatments were in Beverly Hospital. Unfortunately, she did not survive, and that was very hard for me.

When stuff like that happens and you are already very vulnerable, it makes you wonder what your purpose is here in this thing we call life. As I've learned, you have to be positive because life is short. Find the hidden message in your journey, whether it be good or not so much!

"Although the world is full of suffering, it is also full of the overcoming of it."
~ Helen Keller

Chapter 6

To Hair or Not to Hair?

♥

> "Beauty is no quality in things themselves:
> It exists merely in the mind which
> contemplates them; and each mind
> perceives a different beauty."
> ~ David Hume

My Great Worry

One of the very first questions that I remember thinking and asking the medical team about was based on my awareness of cancer patients: "Am I going to lose my hair?" I nearly fell into depression when the answer was in the affirmative, "Yes, you are going to lose your hair due to the chemotherapy."

Since my hair has always been curly and not very thick, it made it easy to twirl. I had always been a hair twirler since childhood. In fact, I couldn't even remember any moment of my life when I was not twirling my hair, so the thought of not being able to twirl my hair was almost paralyzing at that moment, especially with knowing what I was going to have to deal with.

"What am I going to do? I am a hair twirler!" It was a big part of my identity, and it was saddening to be losing that part of myself. For me, losing my hair was far more than the beauty aspect but included everything else that went along with that. I could only hope that it would just be for a little while until the treatments were done and my hair could grow back.

In the meantime, the doctors suggested that I should look into acquiring a wig. I had never been in need to wear a wig and consequently never needed to shop for one, so the thought of getting a wig for the first time was an interesting occurrence.

Shopping for a Wig

The extent of my wig-shopping and wig-wearing experience to date was pretty much zero, well, unless you count finding a witchy wig or punk rocker's string wig to wear at Halloween time! Besides that, I had never been a person to wear accessories on my head. My initial fear was that wearing a wig would be like wearing a hat, which would just result in me feeling hot and sweaty. I never really wore hats because the hot, sweaty feeling would in turn flatten my hair against my head, and then I would literally be a hot, sweaty mess with a bad hairdo!

First, I had to begin by figuring out, "How am I going to get a wig?" My doctor told me that my health insurance covers wigs, so he told me to call my company for the details. When I made the necessary call, the insurers told me how much they covered and where to buy a wig. I soon found out that there were not very many places specialized to take insurance for cancer patients needing wigs. In fact, there was only one wig shop near me that fit this criteria, so I called up and made an appointment just like one would do before going to a regular hair salon.

At my wig consultation, the lady hairstylist who also worked as a cashier at the shop helped me find a wig. I remember trying out various wigs that piqued my interest, but each time, the lady who was helping me said that those choices wouldn't work for me because they didn't fit me well. I hadn't even tried them on, so I secretly questioned if her input was based on her experience or if she was racist, just didn't want to deal with me or my hairstyle, and wanted to move on to the next person.

"Well, she is the expert, I guess," was my thought at the time.

My idea of a perfect wig was similar to my natural hair since I wanted to look as normal as possible with my curly hair. On the other extreme, I always had the perspective to go big or go home! So, knowing that I was about to lose my hair, I made sure to run out and get a cute little hairdo that I adored and otherwise wouldn't have been brave enough to do had my circumstances been otherwise.

I always dreamed about having a long, voluptuous, curly wig like a princess in a fairy tale. This idea was born when I was younger and went to great lengths to pretend that I had long and flowing hair. As a child, I always chose outfits for Halloween that came with long hair. For example, I liked dressing up as a witch with a long wig, even though the hair was matted. There was even a season where I dressed up as a punk rocker with long, foily hair or cut up t-shirts!

My desire for long hair was in contrast to how my dad used to keep my hair cut short. It started when I was really small from the ages of three to six when my dad parted my hair to the side while calling me his little boy. My aunt would help me by putting a little barrette in my hair when it was short, since I didn't want a boy's hairdo. As my hair grew longer, I would ask my aunt to fix my hair since no one else wanted to comb it or help me take care of it. My dad even had someone come over to the house to cut my hair. When I was about twelve or thirteen, I was so annoyed that I couldn't have long hair, so I started making my own inventions. I began cutting up old tee shirts all the way from the bottom up to the neck band and then wearing them like it was my own long hair.

As I was going through the process of trying on and buying new wigs at the wig shop, I still had my natural hair. In the back of my mind, I kept thinking about how I was going to look in my new wigs once I did lose my hair, since I knew that I was going to look and feel different when it all happened. I found it to be an overwhelming process. I thought, "Just get me something that I like, even if it's not my dream."

The hairstylist and I eventually settled on a wig that was a bobbed style with little bangs, which

I thought would be cute, a bit of a throwback to when bobs were popular. The wig that I settled for cost around $500, which was very expensive at that time! I couldn't believe that the insurance covered $400 for the wig, leaving me to cover the rest of the cost. I also felt like I was forced to go to a specific wig shop and look for certain styles because there were no other options available. Yet, since I didn't have much choice for wigs, why bother sulking in my own misery? As I learned, the whole process is insensitive to cancer patients, even though the way it is set up is probably just trying to make you feel better.

For me, the whole experience made the hair trauma from my younger days resurface. So, I decided to share the situation I just went through with a friend who knew more about wigs than I did. She immediately took me to a small wig store that, in comparison to the first one I had been to, was wonderful! It had a variety of beautiful wigs that I could choose from, and the price difference was also significant: $60 for a nice wig instead of $500 for one that I didn't care much for!

My friend bought a wig for me, and I bought two. These were all dark with longer hair, and one had red highlights. While they weren't quite as long and wavy as my dream fairy tale style, some were close to it! Once my insurance was all set, I went and picked up the bobbed wig, bringing me to a total of four wigs. I felt much happier with my wig situation taken care of.

Farewell, Hair

The way I lost my hair was quick and dramatic. After my first chemo treatment, I was still holding onto my hair, but after the second, it began to be too much. Every time I ran my hands through my hair, I would have chunks of hair in my hands. It started off not being a lot, just a few strands here and there, but gradually increased to a point where I did not want to wait until it all fell out.

I would wake up every morning with 20, 30, or 50 strands of hair piling up on my pillow. Then I would take a shower, wash my hair, wet my hair, and even comb it. There were so many more strands coming out that it was traumatic. I didn't even want to touch my hair at all anymore!

Then there were the hair twirling woes where I would go from feeling soothed to feeling sad. It was like when a river starts to overflow, the dam breaks, and you say, "Oh no!" You actually think that you're going to wake up and find yourself bald one day without realizing that hair loss is a gradual, torturous, slow, painful change when it starts happening.

One early morning before he opened his barber shop for the day, I went to *mi primo hermano*'s who was very close to me. Since it was just so depressing for me as an avid hair-twirler to witness my hair falling out, I just had him shave the rest of my hair. It was a private time, and I had a photographer present also to remember the moment.

With my hair now gone, the stress of when and how it would come off was also gone. It was just nice to have a clean, bald head after the painful process of slowly losing my hair. Now, I just had to learn to look at and appreciate my new normal for the meantime.

The Good, the Bad, and the Ugly

The only question I was left with was, "Now, what will I do with this head?" I began working with my wigs and scarves, figuring out what I'd wear each day based on what things matched. It was a lot to handle day-to-day, knowing that you're looking at yourself in the mirror and trying to look your best. You now have no hair, which is part of your identity and sexuality, but you have the hope that this is only a temporary issue.

I started wearing wigs, and even though it was a rough start, I eventually got used to them. I had never tolerated any garments on my head, be it hats, scarves, or any ornaments, since I would get hot, which turned into me being sweaty. Now that circumstances had forced me to wear wigs, I had to get used to them. I remember that one of the wigs in particular looked good, and I would get compliments from my friends and colleagues whenever I wore it.

On the other hand, I soon became the butt of jokes with a certain other wig, the bob from the first shop I went to. It all began when one person, probably meaning well but definitely not thinking about my feelings, remarked, "You look like Dora with that wig!" Then, suddenly, everyone was calling me Dora. While some thought it was fun and tried to make light of my situation, my feelings would often get hurt. Given that the wig that made me look like Dora was the most expensive wig I had obtained, I realized that it was a very expensive way to be associated with Dora!

The other part of that unfunny situation was that I struggled with my weight since childhood and saw myself as chubby for most of my life. Being called Dora just crushed any remaining self-esteem! It always painted a picture of a fat Dora in my head, and then I would think, "That is me." As a result, I avoided looking at the pictures of me wearing the "Dora the Explorer Wig," and I also did not wear that wig very often.

As I thought about my hair loss and wig situation overall, I felt that not being able to have my dream type of hair via a wig was just adding insult to injury! At the same time, I was happy that my friend was there to help me get something better than the terrible bob. I could face disappointment on so many other levels, but getting a bad hairdo just made it worse. If I had to go back, I would only get what I wanted. That was one of the little things that no one told me about ahead of time, so I had to find it out for myself.

Speaking of chemotherapy, hair loss, and other things they neglect to inform you about is that you will lose *Every. Single. Piece.* of hair on your body, not just on your head. For starters, you lose your eyebrows and take on a different look. As I discovered, wearing a wig with no eyebrows is a peculiar look!

Then, there goes the protective hair in your nose and ears, the fine hair on your arms and legs, and even the hair between your buttocks. Those are the hairs that you don't realize have a purpose until they are gone! Your skin becomes sticky with no hair, and everything becomes a chore. When you put your clothes on, it's a whole long sticky ordeal because you lose the gliding mechanism provided by your body hairs. When you poop, it's no longer a smooth wipe, but becomes an issue to clean yourself. Like, you don't want little crumplets of toilet paper all up in your stuff! You suddenly become aware of what an important role those tiny hairs play!

Between the loss of hair on my head, the loss of hair on my entire body, and the wig complications, I often contemplated just resigning myself to staying home and rocking the bald look anyway. More often, I basically ended up wearing head scarves, which were more comfortable and did not make me feel like I was wearing something heavy on my head. In addition, scarves were also convenient as they matched well with different outfits, and I wasn't being called Dora.

Another reason that I left the wigs behind is that they were very conspicuous. When you have one on, everybody knows you have one on—or at least, so I thought. I always had to pay attention to the lining of the wig and if it was going to match everything perfectly. I had other things to look out for, too. Does the skin color match my natural tone? If I parted my hair, would it look like my scalp color? How far down should the wig rest on my forehead? All of these details come into play when you are wearing a wig, which you wouldn't think about if you're not a wig-wearer!

In fact, my experiences helped me develop a mindset of intuition over the years where I've been able to pinpoint things that I previously did not notice. For example, if someone's been very overweight and lost a lot of weight naturally or through surgery, I can usually tell. Also, to a certain degree, I can tell if someone is in the earlier stages of cancer and wearing a wig. These were things that I didn't think about and couldn't recognize until I had my own situation.

Welcome Back, Hair!

After the chemo treatments were over, my hair finally started to grow back. Thank goodness! *¡Gloria a Dios, por fin!* I noticed that dressing and other daily tasks gradually became easier. The hair on my head changed texture from what it was originally, being a lot thinner and wavier rather than thicker and curlier.

I was especially happy to be able to start playing with my hair again, which was something I hadn't done for a very long time. Seeing my hair begin to grow in and being able to twirl my new locks was a small bit of relief in dealing with a number of other things that I would have to face for the rest of my life.

Meanwhile, I waited patiently for my eyebrows to grow fully in and... they never did! At first, when my eyebrows started growing back, they were so thin that I thought they were "still coming in" for a long time. I struggled with how thin they were, and I still do. There was nothing I could do to change things, but I was simply grateful to have my hair back! As it grew back,

I rocked a hairstyle that was shaved short on one side and longer on the other, and I loved it!

> "In the deepest slumber
> No! In delirium
> No! In a swoon
> No! In death
> No! Even in the grave
> All is not lost."
> ~ Edgar Allan Poe

Chapter 7

Ringing the Bell

♥

"What we call a new beginning is often the end. And to make an end is to make a beginning. The end is where we start from."
~ T.S. Eliot

The Bell

When going for my radiation treatments at MGH, I noticed a bell at the end of the hallway of the breast cancer treatment center. It hung there, prompting my curiosity, and I soon learned that it was there to signify and celebrate the successful completion of each patient's ordeal. I also saw a few people ringing the bell during my appointments there and was able to congratulate them for successfully completing their treatments.

I couldn't wait for my turn! It was a small token that helped me stay hopeful and start my countdown. I looked forward to the point where I could take a break from all of the exhausting appointments and finally get my life back.

Once I finally reached the point where it was my turn to ring the bell, I came to realize that my treatments were actually not quite over. It just meant that a major part of the journey in receiving the initial treatments was over, and it was time to step into a new phase. And just like that, I had my last radiation treatment and was met by my team at THE BELL.

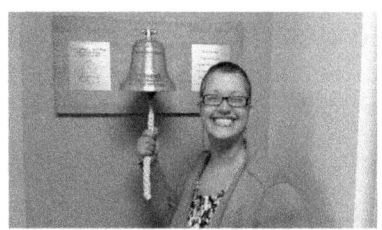

IT WAS FINALLY MY TURN TO RING THE BELL!

Ahh, that was satisfying! I was finally on to the next phase!

The next thing that happened was that the doctor and medical team set me up on a medicine course for the next several years. This was standard, and the course was supposed to last for five to ten years, depending on the type of breast cancer each person was diagnosed with.

As I came to grips with this new phase, I also learned firsthand about the many lasting symptoms from chemotherapy and radiation that I had to deal with. Unfortunately, I had already developed very bad neuropathy since the beginning, which was a huge symptom for many patients. And don't forget my horrible experience with kidney stones! Yet, I mistakenly thought that everything would end following the dreadful hair loss.

Tamoxifen

My type of breast cancer was estrogen-positive, which meant that I would need to be put on a medication called Tamoxifen for at least five years. According to breast cancer research, when taking 20mg of Tamoxifen every day for up to ten years, this drug is an effective treatment in preventing the recurrence of cancer.

I am not a person who likes to take medications, and I tend to avoid as many kinds of manufactured pills and artificial remedies as possible. Thus, the thought of taking medications every day for at least five to ten years was a little unsettling! Plus, I was not used to taking a daily pill of any sort, so when I began taking the prescribed 20mg of Tamoxifen, there were many days that I forgot to take the daily dosage.

Then there were the many side effects! The worst was the night sweats. I began to sweat profusely at night and would often wake up drenched in my own sweat. This resulted in me not sleeping well most of the time and went on for months on end, which was very difficult to deal with.

When I first mentioned it to the doctors, they wondered if I had an early onset of menopause, since that could be one of the effects, so testing was done! I explained my symptoms on numerous occasions when at the doctors, especially my sleeping problems and generally not feeling so great since being on Tamoxifen. Every time I talked to the doctors about it, they offered to give me a prescription to deal with the side effects. Although I was suffering, the last thing I was going to do was to take more pills to help treat side effects caused by the original medication that I was taking!

I told the doctor, "Never will I ever take a new prescription to deal with the side effects of the original medication!" I was adamant about not taking anything extra for the side effects and decided that I would stop taking Tamoxifen altogether before I took additional prescriptions.

My doctor was empathetic toward my concerns and decided to reduce the Tamoxifen dosage from 20mg to 10mg. As a result, the night sweats I was experiencing decreased significantly, finally allowing me to sleep much better. I chose to stay on that lower dose and took it every morning, which was part of my daily routine for the last ten years.

Am I Cancer-Free?

Every time I visited the doctor for a follow-up, I was always filled with reserved optimism. I nervously waited for his updates about the status of the cancer, and I would have loved for the doctor to tell me, "You are now cancer-free!" However, I knew the truth: after undergoing chemotherapy, surgery, and radiation, sometimes the cancer cells go into remission but could still recur later on.

What a tough pill to swallow, especially while undergoing everything else! It is so difficult to face this uncertainty, knowing that a positive outcome is not really known and thus not guaranteed. Yet, we all must keep our heads up and do the best we can by continuing to eat a healthy diet and exercise regularly.

As I discovered, doctors never come out and say, "You're cancer-free!" The only straightforward thing that I did hear from them was at the very beginning of my ordeal, "You have cancer." Later on, after the initial treatment and checking my lymph nodes to a certain depth to see if the cancer spread, the doctor told me, "The tumor is gone, and the margins are clear."

I had to do my own research to find out what that meant and why doctors say things in the way they do. In so many words, it all comes down to this: we all have cancerous cells, and cancer can appear in us anywhere and at any time. So, the reality is, I could be cancer-free in the initial area where the problem was discovered, but something else could be developing somewhere else in my body. I could walk out and be breast cancer-free free but have it somewhere else.

So, as I discovered, doctors never say, "You're cancer-free!" to avoid malpractice. At the same time, I think that their explanation could be a lot clearer and offer more comfort to cancer patients who go through so much of a painful ordeal. Perhaps, if the doctor's office provided a brochure or some other kind of information, it would shift the conversation away from that uncertain talk about margins and better explain, "The main threat is resolved."

My Lifestyle Changes

I knew from the very beginning that my lifestyle prior to my diagnosis was something I needed to adjust. I especially needed to make some changes to my dietary choices. When I met with the doctors early on, I remember him saying that diet can be implicated in the diagnosis and prognosis. Eating fatty and greasy takeout, no matter how tasty, needed to stop. The same went for frozen and processed foods, so fruits and veggies it was!

At the same time, let's be real: developing and keeping healthy habits is really hard! We shouldn't beat ourselves up or be too judgmental when everything doesn't go according to our healthy plan. After all, the negative self-appraisal is even worse than eating McDonald's because it takes a toll on us mentally. You ate the French fries when you knew they weren't really healthy for you? Oh well, I did, too. We can do better next time, and still be kind to ourselves. Maybe it's time to go for a brief walk!

As the years passed following my initial treatments, I could see how easy it is to forget the minor details of your cancer journey over time. Many memories became fuzzy except for the most significant and traumatic moments of the treatment journey: the trauma of going to appointments, getting sick to your stomach, not being able to eat whatever you want, and other horrible things like that.

Following chemo, whenever I ate, many things tasted like metal. I found that even water had a bad taste, so I usually drank lemonade and water that tasted like lemon. I was told that I should try ginger candies, but they were gross! I also heard that smoothies were a good option, so I started making an easy smoothie every day. They were the best—until they weren't. One day, I suddenly needed to throw up, and it was so bad with all this yogurt consistency that I realized my body had never really digested all the smoothies I had enjoyed! From then on, it was back to lemon water, lemonade, and occasionally smoothies without yogurt.

Besides what I've already mentioned, there were other side effects and after-effects from the cancer treatment: sharp pains in my breast, pains in my feet, physical weakness that took time to get back to normal, and more. My body was very weak for a long time, and I even suffered a torn meniscus in my knee after an overly excited student gave me a big hug, accidentally knocking me down and causing the injury. The irony was that it was the very last day of school, and I just bought roller blades the weekend prior so I could build my strength and BOOM!

The major part of dealing with cancer that I remember was facing daily activities of living—without ease. Whether it was struggling with small, normal things at home or interacting with people outside the home, there was added difficulty to each part of life.

Yet, life after cancer has its challenges as well. Sometimes, it's an unexpected memory that takes me by surprise. Not too long ago, for instance, I visited a friend in the hospital and had a semi-flashback of going through cancer treatments. As I've been in hospital scenarios a few times now, I know that this is a normal part of the process of dealing with memories that pop up now and then.

Other times, the challenge comes when meeting acquaintances or casually bumping into others when out and about, such as people who knew you when you were first diagnosed and going through the treatment ordeal. They often say, "Oh, how are you doing?" with a look of pity and sympathy. You can tell that they are wondering whether you are still on treatments and how you are faring.

While it happened much more frequently at the beginning, even after the treatments are long over, I still notice that I get looks whenever I run into certain people. Of course, I understand where they are coming from, but each interaction reminds me of where I once was and makes me feel bad for a moment because it brings up those old memories to reflect on. It's much different facing these people compared to the friends you see all the time, because the people who know you well know how you're doing today, but not everyone has that insight.

As the years continue to pass, bumping into people who only knew me from that time in my life causes an awkward interaction. "Oh, you look well," they will say. Even though it's been ten years, it reminds me how time moves both slow and fast. While I thought all of that was over and behind me, that's the only thing they remember about me! Such moments help me be more cognizant of others, since a tragedy or trauma doesn't define someone for the rest of their lives, even though that might be the only thing I know or remember about them.

The whole experience also gave me a new recognition for others who are going through cancer, partly because I could see the after-effects on their body and partly from a sense of intuition in having been there myself. You notice it because of the amount of trauma and changes that the body goes through for an extended period of time. Also, when people are going through treatment, you can immediately tell that as well, especially when they are wearing a wig or head scarf.

Old Endings and New Beginnings

Before it was my turn to ring the bell, I kept the District Attorney informed about how my cancer treatment was progressing. Once everything was over in the middle of November, I told their office that it was time to resume the trials. This was the other heavy, negative thing in my life that I was eager to see come to an end! Just a few short weeks later, we had the trial. By the end of the year, the judgment was back, and everything was finally over.

As January and the New Year arrived, I felt that everything was behind me and that I could try and recover with my life back to normal. I already had the feet of a new teacher, which didn't free up any time but did reduce a lot of stress. After all, the expenses that I faced in all of these situations were extreme, so I knew that I needed to continue working and advancing my career.

At the same time, teaching became another thing to worry about. As soon as the cancer treatments were over, I wondered if I would be able to get my master's in the allotted time or if I could somehow come up with money to get into Class Measures to advance my license. I kept a pretty hopeful attitude that I would accomplish a lot of things in a short amount of time and found a master's degree program starting in September that allowed me to study full-time for two years while working full-time and still recovering.

I was happy to get back on track in completing my education and pushed through to finally receive my master's. How happy and proud I was to walk across the stage to receive my certificate!

More Heartache

The day after graduation, however, tragedy struck. I lost my mom after her own battle with pancreatic cancer. Immediately, I was sent into a tailspin of sadness and reflection about how much I needed and missed her in my life.

My mom and I had a wonderful relationship, but it was an odd one. Because I didn't live with her the whole time I was growing up, we didn't see each other all the time. I spoke to her weekly and saw her about once a month, sometimes more and sometimes less. We were both fine with this.

As we grew older, my mom and I grew closer. I shared many things with her and even invited her out to enjoy all kinds of shenanigans with us, from birthday dinners to walks. Even though she declined many of my invitations, I knew it meant a lot to my mom that I was including her in my daily activities.

My mom was always proud of my accomplishments, and beating cancer was no different. She also knew I was under a lot of pressure to finish my schooling so I could continue teaching. My first year of school wasn't so bad, so I stayed in very close contact with her and saw her a lot.

I wish I could say the same of my second year, but that one was drastically different, especially my last semester of school. I got so caught up in my education that I didn't realize how much we had drifted apart. In fact, my eyes were bulging with so much school work that I didn't even recognize how much time was going by without me seeing her! All I knew was that I had deadlines and needed to graduate.

The last semester was especially the hardest. I also met my boyfriend during that year and was trying to juggle a new relationship. In fact, that April, my mom met him, and I privately shared with her, "I think I love my boyfriend, but I haven't said anything to him yet." In response, Mom told me to tell my boyfriend the truth if that was how I really felt. I was so glad to have her advice and support!

The next month was May, and the pressure was on to finish everything before graduation! I hung up lists all over my house with things that had to be done within the month in order for me to graduate.

One day when I was in the shower, I suddenly felt the intuition that I was going to lose someone. I immediately began crying, thinking that it might be Mama, my grandmother, because she was old and in hospice.

At one point, I reached out to my mom to tell her how I think I managed to pull everything off and meet all the last deadlines, but it was hard for me to get in touch with her. Finally, I texted her about my graduation and was happy to get her response that she said she would go. I also told her that I was trying to be the commencement speaker, and that it was between me and just one other person. As always, Mom told me that she was proud of me!

Unfortunately, my mom never made it to my graduation. My intuition was correct that I was going to lose someone—except that it wasn't Mama. Instead, it was my mom!

> **"Every new beginning comes from some other beginning's end."**
> **~ Seneca**

Epilogue

♥

Reconstructive Surgery?

Even after everything that I have been through and seeing myself as such a fighter, it is still hard to look in the mirror and see my uneven breasts. Following the end of my treatment, I became, and still am, very self-conscious.

Prior to my breast cancer diagnosis, I always had small breasts, but it was never something I worried about. Now, I look at my breasts in the mirror, and it makes me want to cry. Not only does it worsen my self-consciousness, but it also drains my self-esteem. The breast that had cancer is smaller than the other and has a noticeable dent in it, and my breasts look lopsided when viewed together. If I lean over, the difference is even more glaring and bothers me to the high heavens.

With each new length of time in my recovery, I had to learn to become more comfortable with different things that arose in my life because my appearance was such a grief to me. For example, after the first several years, I was able to get back on birth control. Then, as my hair grew in, I started playing with different hairstyles to see if any of them would be more appealing to me than others.

In the summer, when it was warm enough to wear a bathing suit or low-cut shirts, I was very self-conscious about how my breasts looked.

When exercising, if any cleavage was showing, I'd wear a little cover-up to hide scarring and abnormalities. It really bothered me at first, but as enough time passed over the years, it both grew on me and prompted me to do something different.

During a physical in the past year, I finally asked my doctor about reconstructive surgery. After making an appointment with the specialist, I had the option to start the process by setting up a couple of consultations. I provided a whole list of questions that I was concerned about getting the right answers to:

Will I get implants?

What's the risk with that?

Should I settle for what I have now?

Should I not settle because it's my body, and I want to look my best?

Let's be real: when it comes down to it, it's not a big deal for me about how people look at me. Instead, it's how I look at myself! In that sense, I thought about having reconstructive surgery frequently, hoping that it would be yet another step where I'll be able to heal from and overcome the traumatic experience that I went through.

Of course, I realize that cancer is not an experience that I'll ever forget. Sometimes, the memories are heavier than at other times. Occasionally, I find myself looking at things differently, such as when I check food ingredients and analyze them with a whole new lens. I hope that getting reconstructive surgery will at least ease my self-conscious mindset and make me more confident in myself.

So, ten years after my treatment was over, it was finally time to meet with a reconstructive surgeon. First, he asked me why I waited so long, upon which I shared that I tend to wait a long time for many things and wanted to make sure I was fully healed—not only in the surgery and tissue but physically and emotionally as well.

Once we established that I was interested in knowing options for asymmetry, he told me right away that, due to radiation, implants were 100% off the table. The only way asymmetry could be achieved was by adjusting the form of my good boob, or the one that did not have the cancer.

Being no fool, I knew that having some cosmetic surgery while under the knife at a discounted rate sounded appealing, but that was also something I could do without the reconstructive surgery. At the same time, I am not going to lie, I was pretty devastated.

Did I make the wrong choice in the original lumpectomy? I wanted a nice implant to round out and fix my "sick" boob, but that was not an option. Meanwhile, the thought of touching the boob that was never affected made me sad. As an original part of me that has never been touched, damaged, infected, or changed except for natural gravity, if I made changes to it, I would never know what my breasts would have looked like naturally when I am older.

At the same time, if I did address the asymmetry, would it help things look better as I age? I could only imagine that the operated boob will stay on the firmer side, and the non-operated one will continue to change with gravity.

When I factored in not having my mom around any longer, I decided that I probably won't go with the surgery. I still need my mom, not only for the decision but for the recovery. Since she is not here, I most likely will not go through with it. Writing the book without her was hard enough, and yet, I still know that she is proud of me for what I have accomplished in my healing journey.

Looking Toward a Bright Future

In looking back over my journey and forward to the future, there are some things that I prefer not to remember and a lot of other things that I don't want to forget. Whenever I try to ignore what happened, it puts a little depression on me, like I'm hiding something big in a little black box and it's a jack-in-the-box, just waiting to pop out in an ugly and scary way.

Instead, having faced and successfully overcome cancer, I accept it as a big part of who I am and how I look at things through a different lens today. Even when I see my own shortcomings, such as where diet is concerned, I can embrace the trauma that has happened and has made me who I am now. Best of all, I have the understanding of what it takes so I can be there for others, which is a big part of who I am!

One big thing that happened more recently was that I successfully weaned myself off of Tamoxifen. I realized that it was a crutch for me, since I subconsciously thought of it as a cure-all and that cancer couldn't return while taking that medication. The reality was, however, that I had to stop taking it, and the doctor only allowed me a few extra months of the "crutches."

During the time of weaning myself off of Tamoxifen, I made time solely for the purposes of my health and well-being. Once again, it was important to keep my mind busy instead of allowing it to go to a dangerous place.

I was not warned of any side effects of stopping Tamoxifen, and I didn't give it much thought UNTIL I got my period and bled for like two months! I looked it up online and found out that it was normal. Yet, what was really odd was not just getting my period again but also how I felt—like my old self again in a very hormonal way. For instance, I would go from crying to laughing in the drop of a dime if the situation was right. My emotions were running wild, and I thought, "Wow, that part is over now, too!"

Once I successfully finished taking the Tamoxifen, that concluded any and all breast cancer things medically. Going forward, I only need to keep up with yearly mammograms, which is also very scary every single time you get one, due to the dense tissue created by the surgery to remove the tumor.

Despite any of the ongoing challenges that I face, I am looking forward to the next chapter in my life. Writing this book allowed me to heal in deeper ways than I could have ever imagined I needed. I've found healing not only from my cancer story, what I went through, and continue to struggle with, but also from the grief of my mom's passing away.

Although I will never fully and truly heal from the loss of my mother, I am able to acknowledge my feelings more. For example, I remember certain aspects like how things ended with my schooling, how she was not there for my graduation, how she was sick, and how I've felt like I never showed her how much I really appreciated her. Throughout all of these things, I am looking forward to focusing on my health, healing from other trauma, and exploring the new creative writing side of me.

Life is short, so why not give it a try?!

Follow the Author

♥

Thank you for joining me as I shared my beautiful mess with breast cancer! Let's not part ways just yet—feel free to reach out to me anytime through any of my links or details below.

Most of all, if you found anything in my story that resonated with your own journey and the stresses and struggles that you have faced, **Please Leave a Book Review!**

Author Page on Substack:
https://substack.com/@amandafeliz

Facebook:
https://www.facebook.com/afeliz1 or search "Amanda Tink Happy Feliz"

Instagram:
https://www.instagram.com/tinkfeliz or search "Amanda Tink Happy Feliz"

TikTok:
https://www.tiktok.com/@amanda.tink.happy.feliz

Email:
Feliz_auth@proton.me

Snail Mail:
Amanda Feliz
PO BOX 2623
Lynn, MA 01903

Practical Tips from an Overcomer

♥

Tips for Cancer Patients

DURING TREATMENT

Get sunlight if possible.

Wear all things comfortable and soft.

Take warm showers and baths.

Drink lots of water. Also, find other drinks like lemonade to keep flavors flowing on the tongue.

Eat hard candy like ginger drops.

Drink tea.

Keep healthy mini meals and snacks on hand. Baked snacks are especially good for crunch, flavor, and health.

Enjoy your favorite hobby to stay busy, or maybe take the time to try out and learn a new hobby like crocheting, painting, arts and crafts, or gardening.

Read books.

Do crossword puzzles, sudoku, and word search to keep your mind occupied. L

Journal and spend time in self-reflection. Allow yourself to acknowledge and feel your emotions. If you need to have a good cry or laugh, be gentle to yourself and do it!

Find support from other people who are also dealing with cancer. Maybe this means finding someone you know to talk to or joining a support group, but discussing the journey with someone who has been in the same shoes is very helpful.

AFTER CANCER CARE

Start with the basics: take walks and then move into strength training and cardio. Get that body moving!

Rest a lot and sleep as much as you can.

Eat healthy! Healthier eating will improve your overall health. As far as cravings go, I say that if you want something and it's not good for you, don't eat it right away. Instead, pay attention to the craving and your emotions that you are feeling. Try to distract yourself for ten minutes with a hobby, your favorite show, or taking a walk. If time has passed and you still want it, then EAT IT! Do not deprive yourself, and do not feel guilty!

Focus on stress management with personal care. For example, get your nails done or do them yourself on a regular basis, sign up for massages, explore new things, and learn a new hobby or perfect an old one.

Be kind to yourself. Be gentle, allow emotions to come and go when they arise, and pay attention to your body.

If you do these things, when you least expect it, you will be feeling and looking better than you have in a long time!

Tips for Friends and Family Who Want to Support

Call to check in and say hi, even if that means leaving a voice message or sending a text instead. There are never too many messages! Just be okay with your call or text possibly not being returned.

Stop by to say hi.

Offer to go grocery shopping.

Drop off meals.

Offer time for their children to be out of the home, if they have younger kids.

Mail or deliver cards and notes of encouragement.

Send or drop off flowers.

Put together small tokens to let them know you are thinking of them.

Organize group gatherings in their honor.

Fundraise for expenses if possible.

Offer to keep them company when they're lonely at home or when they need someone to go with them to appointments or treatments.

Give gifts to keep them mentally occupied, like books to read or things that go with their favorite hobby. Another great present is gift cards for food.

Acknowledgments

♥

I want to give a very big thank you and a huge shoutout to everyone who was very supportive, helping me get through this illness and looking out for me during my journey!

To my mom (may she rest in peace), who was at every chemo appointment and more.

To my son, who kept me company on the way to appointments and at home. Without his innocence, joy, and humor, I would have been miserable! (Calliou)

To Lynn Shore Little League, thank you for keeping my son busy! My son was playing baseball at the time, and there were a few coaches who would bring him home after practice so I wouldn't have to go out, and they also made sure he made it to the games!

To the staff at the elementary school I worked at, you are a special group, and your support was more than I could ask for.

To the few ladies who went out with me the night I found out my devastating news.

To my Big C Sistah, Maria, we'll always have each other's backs!

To Maleeka, for teaching me how to crochet! I relied heavily on it during my treatments.

To Debbie Brown and her friend Holly, for keeping my after-school crochet group afloat. Also, to the crochet group, who continued making squares when I couldn't.

To Elizabeth Crowley-Burns, the meal plan was the best! Thank you to all the people who signed up and brought me food! It was a huge weight lifted off my shoulders! Liz, thank you also for taking Wes out on a few occasions. From paint night to camping, you made a child worry a little less, be more of a kid, and have fun!

To my cousin Michael, who cut my remaining hair off.

To Jay, for taking some pictures of me.

To Elizabeth H., for really helping this book come to light. So glad we found you!

AND the biggest acknowledgement to *Mi Amor*, Nicholas. This book would not have been possible without you! Although you weren't there when I had my battle because I met you a few years later, you have been a true believer in me. You've not only motivated, encouraged, and helped me write my story, but you've also provided me with all the support I needed during each and every step of the book-writing journey and in facing all the healing that has come out of it. There were a lot of emotions and support, so a simple "Thank you" is truly not enough. Words cannot describe my immense gratitude towards you! You are the BEST and have changed my life for the BEST!! I LOVE YOU!!

Resources

♥

Advanced Breast Cancer Community
http://advancedbreastcancercommunity.org/
A comprehensive information source and online community solely dedicated to the needs of advanced/metastatic breast cancer patients, caregivers, family, friends, and healthcare providers.

Breast Cancer Organization
https://www.breastcancer.org/
An organization that provides community and support for breast cancer patients, operating with the goal to offer trusted guidance when it is

needed most, because no one should face breast cancer alone.

Living Beyond Breast Cancer
https://www.lbbc.org/
Living Beyond Breast Cancer is a national, non-profit organization that offers on-demand emotional, practical, and evidence-based content that is meaningful to those newly diagnosed, in treatment, post-treatment, and living with metastatic disease.

Mayo Clinic
https://www.mayoclinic.org/tests-procedures/brca-gene-test/about/pac-20384815
An article about the BRCA gene test for breast and ovarian cancer risk, and how this blood test uses DNA analysis to identify harmful changes or mutations in both the BRCA1 and BRCA2 susceptibility genes.

Metastatic Breast Cancer Network (MBCN)

http://www.mbcn.org/

MBCN strives to help those living with stage IV breast cancer be their own best advocate by providing education and information regarding treatments and coping with the disease.

METAvivor

http://www.metavivor.org/

This website brings public awareness to the issues of metastatic breast cancer and provides support and resources to patients coping with metastatic breast cancer.

Mothers Supporting Daughters with Breast Cancer

http://www.mothersdaughters.org

Provides a communication network, support, and education for mothers whose daughters are fighting breast cancer.

MyBCTeam on Ports
https://www.mybcteam.com/resources/chemo-ports-for-breast-cancer-types-pictures-what-to-expect
This article has a lot of helpful explanatory information and pictures about the placement of a port before receiving chemotherapy.

National Cancer Institute on Radiation
https://www.cancer.gov/about-cancer/treatment/types/radiation-therapy
Informative article, "Radiation Therapy to Treat Cancer," to learn more about this stage of treatment.

National Cancer Institute on BRCA Genes
https://www.cancer.gov/about-cancer/causes-prevention/genetics/brca-fact-sheet
Fact sheet, "BRCA Gene Changes: Cancer Risk and Genetic Testing," to learn more about common questions and answers.

Share

http://www.sharecancersupport.org
Offers self-help, a hotline, and programs for women with breast/ovarian cancer.

Susan G. Komen for the Cure

https://www.komen.org
Provides funding and programs for research, education, screening,and treatment.

Triple Negative Breast Cancer Foundation

http://www.tnbcfoundation.org
The TNBC Foundation was started by a group of young women who have been personally affected by triple negative breast cancer.

United Breast Cancer Foundation

http://www.ubcf.info
This foundation financially supports a variety of programs dedicated to breast cancer screening, prevention, treatment, and patient health and well-being.

About the Author

♥

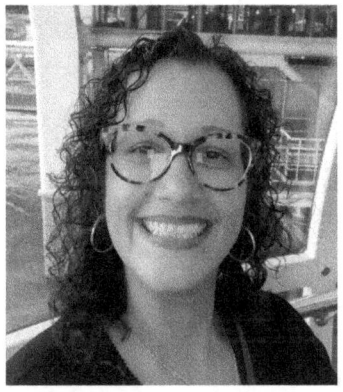

Amanda Feliz is from Lynn, Massachusetts, and finds her tranquility by the ocean. She loves to listen to the ocean sounds, walk the beach, and bike along the shore. Amanda spends her days as an English language educator, being passionate about helping her students find their voices, just like she has found her own in writing.

Amanda lives life with her heart on her sleeve and graciously handles all the surprises life throws her way. As a breast cancer survivor, her resilience is woven into every page she writes. This debut book is inspired by her journey and marks the beginning of the next chapter in her life.

Amanda cherishes time spent with her two adult children, who always inspire her. When time allows, she crochets, teaches Zumba to kids, and travels to wherever her heart desires. She plans on writing more books, including one based on one of the most unbelievable stories that has happened to her, as well as children's stories.

While her world is always filled with many twists and turns, Amanda writes from a place of gratitude, humor, and deep joy. Her words offer laughter, inspiration, and the gentle reminder that even in the darkest moments, life is worth dancing through.